FROZEN DREAMS

FROZEN DREAMS

PSYCHODYNAMIC DIMENSIONS OF INFERTILITY AND ASSISTED REPRODUCTION

edited by

Allison Rosen
Jay Rosen

THE ANALYTIC PRESS

2005   Hillsdale, NJ   London

Published by
The Analytic Press, Inc., Publishers
    Editorial Offices:
    101 West Street
    Hillsdale, NJ 07642

    www.analyticpress.com

Designed and typeset by CompuDesign, Charlottesville, VA

Index by Leonard Rosenbaum, Washington, DC

Library of Congress Cataloging-in-Publication Data

Frozen dreams : psychodynamic dimensions of infertility and assisted reproduction / edited by Allison Rosen, Jay Rosen.
    p. cm.
  Includes bibliographical references and index.
  ISBN 0-88163-383-6 (hc)   0-88163-440-9 (pbk)
    1. Infertility. 2. Infertility—Psychological aspects. I. Rosen, Allison. II. Rosen, Jay.

  RC889.F76 2005
  616.6'92—dc22

                    2004046224

Printed in the United States of America

10 9 8 7 6 5 4 3 2 1

To the fruitful dreams of our mothers, Kay and Ally,
may they multiply in the dreams of our sons, Ben and Sam

CONTENTS

CONTRIBUTORS

Linda D. Applegarth, Ed.D. is Director, Psychological Services at the Center for Reproductive Medicine & Infertility, Weill Medical College of Cornell University, and Assistant Professor of Psychology in the Departments of Obstetrics & Gynecology, Psychiatry, and Reproductive Medicine at Weill-Cornell Medical College, The New York Presbyterian Hospital, New York, NY.

Linda Hammer Burns, Ph.D. is Director, Counseling Services, Reproductive Medicine Center in Minneapolis, MN; Assistant Professor, Department of Obstetrics, Gynecology, and Women's Health at the University of Minnesota Medical School, Minneapolis, MN; and founding member and chair, International Infertility Counseling Organization.

Sharon N. Covington, M.S.W. is Director, Psychological Support Services, Shady Grove Fertility Reproductive Science Center, Rockville, MD; and Assistant Clinical Professor of Obstetrics and Gynecology at Georgetown University School of Medicine, Washington, DC.

Todd Essig, Ph.D. is Supervising Analyst, Supervisor of Psychotherapy, and Fellow, William Alanson White Institute; Clinical Assistant Professor of Psychiatry in Psychology, New York Medical College; founder, and director, Psychoanalytic Connection (psychoanalysis.net); and Chair, Board of Directors, New York Disaster Counseling Coalition (NYDCC).

Nancy Freeman, Psy.D., a clinical psychologist and psychoanalyst with expertise in mother–infant treatment and the experience of infertility and adoption, is on the faculty of the National Institute for the Psychotherapies and the Manhattan Institute for Psychoanalysis.

Dorothy Greenfeld, M.S.W. is Director of Psychological Services, Yale Fertility Center; and Associate Clinical Professor of Obstetrics and Gynecology, Yale University School of Medicine.

Elizabeth A. Grill, Psy.D. is clinical psychologist, Center for Reproductive Medicine and Infertility, and Clinical Instructor of Psychology, Department of Obstetrics and Gynecology, Department of Reproductive Medicine and the Department of Psychiatry, New York Presbyterian Hospital-Weill Medical College of Cornell University.

Maria Jackson, R.N., M.A. is a consultant in private practice in Westfield, NJ, and was formerly Nurse Manager for Reproductive Medicine Associates of New Jersey and Institute for Reproductive Medicine at St. Barnabas Medical Center.

Laura Josephs, Ph.D. is a Clinical Assistant Professor of Psychology in Psychiatry, Weill Medical College of Cornell University and consulting psychologist, Center for Reproductive Medicine and Infertility, New York Presbyterian Hospital.

Judith Kottick, L.C.S.W. is a consultant in private practice in Montclair, NJ.

Shelley Lee, Ph.D. is Director of Psychological Services, New York University School of Medicine Program for In Vitro Fertilization, Reproductive Surgery; and Infertility and Clinical Instructor, Department of Obstetrics and Gynecology, New York University School of Medicine.

Frederick Licciardi, M.D. is Director, Oocyte Donation Program, New York University School of Medicine Program for In Vitro Fertilization, Reproductive Surgery, and Infertility; and Associate Professor, Department of Obstetrics and Gynecology, New York University School of Medicine.

Anne F. Malavé, Ph.D., a clinical psychologist, psychoanalyst, and supervisor, Pace University, specializes in infertility and adoption and is in private practice in Manhattan.

Allison Rosen, Ph.D. (editor) is Supervisor of Psychotherapy, Past President, and Fellow, William Alanson White Institute; Co-Founder of the Fertility Preservation Special Interest Group, American Society of Reproductive Medicine; Medical Advisory Board Member FertileHope; Assistant Editor, *Contemporary Psychoanalysis*.

Jay Rosen (editor) is President, Xint Corp (information technology), and an activist in education and desegregation.

Robert I. Watson Jr., Ph.D. is Supervisor of Psychotherapy, William Alanson White Institute; Adjunct Assistant Professor, Teachers' College, Columbia University; and Staff Psychologist, Columbia-Presbyterian East Side.

ACKNOWLEDGMENTS

This book has been in development for several years and we have many people to thank for their ideas, support, and generous insight. First, we want to acknowledge the many infertile men and women who taught us about the enduring pain, loss of hope, and, most important, the human capacity to be resilient and generative in the face of the deep despair that infertility may entail. Second, we offer our profound thanks to the authors who gave their time, patience, and experience to complete this project.

We acknowledge also the many people at the William Alanson White Psychoanalytic Institute who encouraged and stimulated us; Betsy Hegemen, Ph.D., Jill Bellinson, Ph.D., and Marylou Lionells, Ph.D. deserve special thanks for their vision and friendship.

Members of the RESOLVENYC board, Linda D. Applegarth, Ed.D., Alan S. Berkeley, M.D., Angela Cifone, Ph.D., Karen B. Clarke, Todd Essig, Ph.D., Maria Jackson, R.N., M.A., Isaac Kligman, M.D., Anne Malavé, Ph.D., Christopher Panczner, J.D., Zev Rosenwaks, M.D., Cecilia Schmidt Sarosi, M.D., Stephen Spandorfer, M.D., and Robert I. Watson Jr., Ph.D., gave their time to the infertile community. They encouraged us to find new ways to address the complex needs we all face together when helping our patients achieve their dreams of having children. Diane Aronson, the former executive director of RESOLVE, and Sue Slotnick, the current president of RESOLVENYC, deserve special mention.

The original mental health infertility peer supervision group, including Patricia Mendell, L.C.S.W., Jane Rosenthal, M.D., and Shelley Lee, Ph.D., Robert I. Watson Jr., Ph.D., and Linda D. Applegarth, Ed.D., first established the possibility of multiprogram cooperation and joint effort to reach across professional disciplines and theoretical outlooks. This collaboration served as a seed for this book. The "tristate shrinks," including Kris Bevilacqua, Ph.D., Jennifer Gampers, M.S.W., Dorothy Greenfeld, L.C.S.W., Elizabeth Grill, Psy.D., Laura Josephs Ph.D., Judy Kottick, L.C.S.W., Claudia Pascale, Ph.D., Mindy Schiffman, Ph.D., Lisa Tuttle, Ph.D., Angela Cifone, Ph.D., and Linda D. Applegarth, Ed.D., continued to ask the tough questions and support each other in the face of difficult decisions honestly addressed.

Kutluk Oktay, M.D., Lindsay Nohr Beck, founder of FERTILE HOPE, and Leslie Schover, Ph.D. deserve special praise for their work to help men and women who might become infertile because of medical conditions. Their inspiration and tireless dedication have been a source of intellectual stimulation and hope for the many beneficial uses of ART.

Andrea Vidali, M.D., Nabil Husami, M.D., and the dedicated professionals at American Fertility taught us about tireless, committed, and compassionate patient care.

Paul Stepansky, Ph.D. and Nancy Liguori at The Analytic Press and Donnel B. Stern, Ph.D. helped make our dream a reality, and did so with grace and humor.

Finally, we would like to thank the "viceroys": Sandra Buechler, Ph.D., Mark Blechner, Ph.D., Richard Gartner, Ph.D., John O'Leary, Ph.D., and Robert I. Watson Jr., Ph.D., who taught us that it is possible to know each other intimately for 25 years and still love and respect each other.

INTRODUCTION

*T*his book is about the deep and burning passion of people who will move heaven and earth to create life. Not only is it a report from the front lines of those struggling with infertility, but also a lens into the hearts and minds of those who treat them. It contains dispatches from "embedded journalists" who, in the thick of action, share not only their observations, but also their innermost feelings. We are privileged to share their experiences as well as their answers to the profound questions introduced by changes in contemporary society and by advances in reproductive medicine.

Many of us have the resources to choose when and how we will bear children. This paradox of freedom and choice has ushered in problems: balancing when and how to create our families in order to provide them with the best lives we can. Many couples, because of lack of knowledge about the dangers of delay of childbearing or through misfortune, will become infertility statistics, statistics that reveal only part of the story, the tragedy of infertility.

Infertility strikes 6.1 million people in the United States. This figure represents 10.2 percent of couples in which the woman is of reproductive age, roughly one in ten couples. However, many times this number of people are affected by infertility, among them hopeful grandparents, aunts and uncles, cousins, friends, children yearning for a sibling. Infertility knows no boundaries: individuals and couples of every race, religious background, and financial stratum may face infertility. More than one million couples seek infertility treatment each year. It is important to remember that infertility is both a disease and a life crisis affecting one's life dreams, sense of meaning, sexual functioning, and spontaneity. Infertility may interfere with love, self-esteem, sense of control, and security in one's body and in the world. It can destroy a couple's financial resources.

It is no wonder that infertility patients seek help confronting these emotional crises. Treatment for the emotional aspects of infertility may occur within an existing psychotherapy treatment or cause individuals to seek treatment for the first time. While there are many excellent books describing how to treat infertility medically and emotionally, at present there are few books offering a glimpse into the minds of therapists as they confront the complex choices about life and death (with implications that will continue into the next generation) made in a (sometimes) hasty manner without time to explore the meaning of the choices for those involved. In other words, most current psychotherapy books about infertility treatment address the infertility patient and the infertility patients' emotional dilemmas without considering the effects of these issues on the therapist or the therapeutic process. However laudable these books are, they do not address the psychological issues arising in the therapist and treatment process in a way that illuminates the emotional reactions therapists may experience when facing these complex issues and how these reactions may limit or help psychotherapy. Put simply, infertility counseling arises from the medical model; the patient has problems, the therapist applies techniques to solve these problems. Experienced clinicians know the limitations of such a point of view.

This book is a lens into the hearts and minds of respected mental health professionals as they face the emotional and ethical dilemmas inherent in working with the searing pain and uncertain future of infertility patients. It is a collaboration written with the view that neither theory nor research alone can adequately address the experiences that are commonplace for those who work with the infertile population. Any gathering of clinicians typically leads to a back channel discussion of therapeutic dilemmas: "How would *you* handle such and such?" The heartfelt sincerity and vulnerability of clinicians trying to address the most effective way to handle complex therapeutic experiences is the starting point of this book.

Most of us working with psychotherapy patients find this collaborative oral tradition more satisfying and thought provoking than formal presentations or scientific studies. In an effort to maintain the open and informative nature of these more private, intimate moments, we asked each contributor to write a jargon-free chapter about his or her personal experiences on a difficult topic that we assigned. The authors, many of whom are noted experts and pioneers in the field of infertility, found the task very challenging. To speak about themselves, to come out from behind the curtain of professional expertise, to reveal doubts rather than certainties, to discuss messy decisions under less than optimal circumstances, evoked anxiety. In addition, we chose to highlight the personal, subjective voice of the authors. We wanted the reader to have a first-hand experience in the consulting room, to see how different therapists think, act, and speak; we wanted to highlight each author's unique style. We believe that this diversity of approaches effectively illustrates the intimate nature of therapeutic work and how different therapists are able to create very different, yet meaningful, therapeutic experiences.

Views of transference, countertransference, and the nature of therapeutic action vary in this collection. In some cases, the difficult thoughts and feelings engendered in the therapist are conceived as unwanted intrusions into the therapeutic experience. Other authors view the therapist as a participant in a dyadic system of self and mutual regulation and *use* their feelings (whether wanted or not) as the essential component of change. Some contributors are comfortable with self-disclosure of their innermost thoughts and feelings, in fact, view mutual examination of these perceptions as an essential ingredient of therapeutic work; others remain private and wish to create a "space" for their patients to explore their feelings without being burdened by those of their therapist/counselor. The editors believe that both therapist and patient mutually influence each other and that the clinician who addresses these powerful interactive experiences (whether disclosed or not) can help their patients achieve meaning from confronting the big issues (life and death, hope and despair) that infertility signifies.

In any subjective approach, there is a delicate balance between self-revelation and confession. We believe that the contributors have effectively walked that line. Additionally, the authors wanted to retain the accuracy of their clinical work, but protect the anonymity of their patients. In all cases described in this book, the names have been changed and irrelevant but identifying details have been altered to protect privacy. In some cases, the clinicians worked with their patients to develop a mutually satisfying disguise. However, the clinical issues have not been altered.

The mental health professionals included in this book work in very different contexts, and these environments create different therapeutic issues: evaluation versus treatment; infertility in an ongoing therapy versus therapy expressly for help treating infertility; psychoeducational counseling versus in-depth psychological treatment. In order to be applicable to a broad base of therapists and other infertility specialists, we included therapists working in private practice as well as professionals working in medical settings. We included psychoanalysts, psychodynamic therapists, and the thoughts and research of those from very different clinical backgrounds.

This book is written for psychiatrists, psychologists, social workers, researchers, nurses, physicians and the interested general reader. Mental health professionals with extensive knowledge of psychodynamic theory may learn how to apply their understanding to infertility, medical crises and adoption. Those with experience in infertility counseling may find that broadening their perspectives to include psychodynamic issues clarifies options and helps to achieve more meaningful experiences with their clients.

Linda Hammer Burns bridges the chasm between the researcher and clinician. Through a combination of extensive knowledge of research and lively clinical examples, she provides both the reader unfamiliar with the psychological changes in infertility and the seasoned infertility counselor a comprehensive overview of psychological changes in infertility, including: individual and couple treatment for male factor infertility; infertility complicated by concomitant physical illness or prior mental illness; and infertility and remarriage.

The authors that follow present their perspectives about a variety of special, though common in the infertility world, circumstances. In her chapter, "Therapist Anxiety about Motivation for Parenthood," Laura Josephs, a seasoned psychologist in private practice and in a reproductive program, describes the familiar, dreaded question. When are the patient's bitterness, anger, lack of optimism, and psychopathology extreme enough to disqualify the patient as a candidate for infertility treatment? When should we be concerned and fear for any resulting offspring? How do we constructively handle these difficult emotions in therapy or evaluation?

All too often, the tragic experience of infertility invades the therapist's world. Nancy Freeman, a knowledgeable psychoanalyst with extensive research experience in the world of infant attachment, describes her awkward self-consciousness and revivified anxiety and insecurity upon diagnosis of her infertility. Through subtle countertransference examples, she shows the poignant impact of the analyst's unfulfilled dreams on the therapeutic experience.

Linda Applegarth, a pioneer in the world of infertility and a noted infertility expert, describes her reactions to "individuals and couples, who, with apparently little or no financial restraints, wish to have a child using medical technology in what we consider to be a self-serving and/or ethically questionable way." Her rich clinical examples describe how to work constructively with such difficult emotions as therapist antipathy toward questionable requests for infertility treatment.

What would you do if a virgin, still living with her parents, arrived in your office requesting sperm donation in order to assist her in becoming pregnant? This is one example of the type of the unusual questions facing Judy Kottick in her role as infertility expert in a large reproductive program. With lively and at times hair-raising and heart-rending case studies, she articulates complex ethical questions and her solutions to "gatekeeping" dilemmas in a reproductive program.

Todd Essig, seasoned psychoanalyst and couples therapist, explores how to use the therapist's personal feelings that arise when "previously settled issues about gender, sexual identity, family of origin, personal worth and self-esteem, and the interplay of intimacy and autonomy become problems once again" under the influence of infertility treatment. He provides a helpful theoretical scaffolding for working with couples and explores, with vivid clinical examples, his thoughts on normative couple behavior.

Elizabeth Grill, a recently married young psychologist in a large productive program, describes her experience of the prejudices and questions of staff members and patients who want to know more about her: "Their assumptions often lead to self-doubt about whether or not I can truly grasp the painful significance of their plight without having suffered through infertility myself, which in turn raises fears that I might one day be faced with their same crises." Her chapter puts a face on the single women who choose to become mothers: the young cancer survivor who freezes eggs prior to chemotherapy; the recently widowed young woman who wishes to have a child with her deceased husband's frozen sperm; the young woman who wants to pursue her career and freeze eggs for later use; the woman who has never found "Mr. Right." Her case studies take the reader into the dark thicket of reproductive choices and the resulting maze of ethical complexities.

When the unthinkable happens, when the patient's longed-for baby dies, when the patient suffers multiple miscarriages, what is the therapist to do? Sharon Covington, a nationally known infertility specialist and expert on perinatal loss, shows the reader how she is able to transform these intense losses, losses many therapists would find too painful to work with, into powerful growth, change, and healing. She enters the patients' hearts and shows the reader hers.

What happens when patients who have been traumatized by prior physical or sexual abuse or by horrific disasters experience infertility? Robert I. Watson, an experienced psychoanalyst, enters into this territory and vividly helps the reader with case examples, a conceptual framework for trauma, and a discussion of common countertransference reactions. Thus, he supplies tools to help those most deeply harmed by prior life experiences.

Too often, large infertility programs are unable to follow the outcome of the pregnancies that they help create; patients progress to their obstetricians and do not wish to be reminded of their infertility through later contact by their infertility providers. Fred Licciardi, a world-renowned infertility specialist, and Shelley Lee, a psychologist and infertility specialist in his large reproductive program, examine cases where the pregnancies were terminated despite the couples' desiring babies for a long time, pursuing infertility treatment, and achieving pregnancies through the use of donated eggs and the husbands' sperm. What happened? Could it have been prevented? What can we learn?

Anne Malavé, a psychoanalyst and adoption specialist, takes us into the world of adoption. She provides the reader with knowledge of adoption options, common fears, and the emotional and psychological challenges facing prospective adopters. She provides a welcome balm after sensationalistic media stories about adoption by giving us the facts rather than the horrors. She does not prescribe a formulaic approach. As she says, "I shall try to help therapists become aware of how adoption, as a powerful magnet or blank screen, attracts deep, primitive feelings, projections, and fears, and how it interacts with each person's history and personal psychodynamics."

The last section of the book deals with the roles and responsibilities of infertility providers. The nurse is the point person in most large programs. Patients have the most contact with her, and she delivers both positive and negative news about pregnancy tests. Maria Jackson is a nationally recognized, award-winning nurse who has developed more than one large donor egg program. She describes the unique pressures and emotional reactions of the infertility nurse. She gives the reader an understanding of the emotional battering many nurses experience and discusses how to protect nurses from the deleterious effects of these outpourings.

Dorothy Greenfeld was one of the first mental health workers in the field of reproductive medicine. As a pioneer, she had no prior data on how to perform her role or what her patients needed. In her chapter, she describes changes in the field and her transition from experiencing "breath-taking" excitement through terror and caution to the multitude of complex emotions that are the ordinary fare for the specialist in reproductive medicine.

Together, these chapters provide an understanding of the complex emotions experienced by men and women denied the opportunity to become parents and the effect of these emotions on those wishing to help them. We believe that the therapist in private practice, the infertility specialist, the psychoanalyst, and the general reader will find the cases compelling and the ethical dilemmas they encompass enlightening. The cases tell us about ourselves and reveal the challenges we face in the process of becoming parents. As we experience the terrible losses and joyous gains described in this book, we are forced to evaluate our lives and rethink our relation to what we consider most valuable in life and our relation to love and work, sexuality, reproduction, mortality, and the future.

FROZEN DREAMS

Part I

The Psychological
Burden of Infertility

1

PSYCHOLOGICAL CHANGES IN INFERTILITY PATIENTS

Linda Hammer Burns

A CHILD WITHIN MY MIND . . .

THE CHILD WILL NEVER LIE IN ME

AND YOU WILL NEVER BE ITS FATHER.

MIRRORS MUST REPLACE THE REAL IMAGE

MAKE IT TRUE SO THAT THE GENTLE LOVEMAKING WE DO

HAS POWERFUL PASSION AND A PARENT'S TRUST.

—Elizabeth Jennings

*T*he landscape of human reproduction changed dramatically over the course of the 20th century (see Table 1). Throughout history, the consequence of sexual intercourse has been parenthood—wanted or otherwise—but the 20th century saw the development of both reliable female birth control and extraordinary reproductive innovations. By the beginning of the 21st century, there were nearly 40 ways to have a baby that do not involve sexual intercourse. (Table 2). These possibilities allow couples with fertility problems to have children; in the past, these couples would have been childless. Many of the treatments or the reproductive possibilities are, however, not without significant consequences, sacrifices, financial burdens, and emotional stresses. While medical

Table 1. Timeline of Major Advances in the Diagnosis and Treatment of Infertility over the 20th Century

Year	Above timeline	Below timeline
1904	BBT	
1910	HSG developed	
1913		Sperm–mucus interaction (Huhner) described
1920	CO_2 used to test fallopian tubes	
1929	Laparoscopy popularized in France	
1940s		First description of normal sperm count
1960	Fertility medications introduced	
1970		Microsurgery of fallopian tubes promoted
1978	First IVF baby born in England	
1980s		Operative laparoscopy popularized
1992	ICSI introduced	

Source: Keye (1999).

Table 2. Methods of Reproduction Without Sexual Intercourse

Intravaginal Insemination

1. Intravaginal insemination with husband/partner
2. Intravaginal insemination with ovulation stimulation ovulation induction medication (e.g. clomid)
3. Intravaginal insemination with superovulation induction medications
4. Intravaginal insemination/donor sperm
5. Intravaginal insemination with ovulation induction medication/donor sperm
6. Intravaginal insemination with superovulation induction medications/donor sperm

Intracervical Insemination

7. Intracervical insemination with husband/partner
8. Intracervical insemination with ovulation stimulation ovulation induction medication (e.g. clomid)
9. Intracervical insemination with superovulation induction medications
10. Intracervical insemination/donor sperm
11. Intracervical insemination with ovulation induction medication/donor sperm
12. Intracervical insemination with superovulation induction medications/donor sperm

Intrauterine Insemination

13. Intrauterine insemination with husband/partner
14. Intrauterine insemination with ovulation induction (e.g., clomid)
15. Intrauterine insemination with superovulation induction medication
16. Intrauterine insemination/donor sperm
17. Intrauterine insemination with ovulation induction (e.g., clomid)/donor sperm
18. Intrauterine insemination with superovulation induction medications/donor sperm

Table 2. *(continued)*

In Vitro Fertilization
19. In vitro fertilization with superovulation medications
20. In vitro fertilization/natural cycle

In Vitro Fertilization-Male Factor Related Treatments
21. In vitro fertilization/intracytoplasmic sperm injection (ICSI)
22. In vitro fertilization/microscopic epididymal sperm aspiration (MESA)/ICSI
23. In vitro fertilization/percutaneous epididymal sperm aspiration (PESA)/ICSI
24. In vitro fertilization/testicular sperm extraction (TESE)/ICSI
25. In vitro fertilization/donor sperm

In Vitro Fertilization-Related Procedures
26. Gamete intrafallopian transfer (GIFT)
27. Tubal embryo transfer (TET)
28. Intrauterine embryo transfer (IVF/ET)
29. Frozen embryo transfer
30. In vitro fertilization/donor egg
31. Donor embryo
32. In vitro fertilization/preimplantation genetic diagnosis
33. Assisted hatching

Gestational Carrier/Surrogacy
34. Surrogacy
35. Gestational carrier with husband/partner sperm
36. Gestational carrier/donor sperm
37. Gestational carrier/donor oocyte
38. Gestational carrier/donor embryo

Other
39. Cloning

science has made strides in the diagnosis and treatment of infertility disorders, mental health has learned more about the psychological impact of involuntary childlessness, the short- and long-term consequences of treatment on individuals, marriages, society, and children (Burns and Covington, 1999). Gone are the days when unexplained infertility was attributed to conflicted feelings toward one's mother or ambivalent feelings about motherhood or parenthood.

PSYCHOLOGICAL RESPONSE TO INFERTILITY

Parenthood (probably more than marriage or other milestones of young adulthood) is often experienced as the *real* "entreé" into adulthood. Without it, people typically feel unable to relate to peers, siblings, or parents as equals. As a result, when parenthood is not achieved—and the years drag on in an effort to achieve it—infertile persons typically feel increasingly distressed, and they feel tension in relation to others. In short, infertility is a multidimensional developmental crisis for individuals, marriages, and families.

Infertility is a crisis of physical and psychological proportions affecting the body, sense of self, and relationships with others. It triggers an array of powerful emotions and responses, including attachment and bereavement issues, internal and external conflicts, relationship and social concerns, object relations issues, and emotional vicissitudes. Early responses to infertility are typically shock, disbelief, anger, blame, shame, and guilt. Over time feelings of loss of control, diminished self-esteem, chronic bereavement, anxiety, and depression are common. Patients complain of the pain of being unable to plan or predict the future. They feel that someone else has control of their lives, bodies, or emotions, whether it is their medical caregivers, God, or some other, outside of themselves—the external other.

Over time, infertility affects how people view the world and themselves. The internal self is affected by feelings of inadequacy, self-blame, identity issues, and diminished status or prestige. These feelings may be directed toward the self or toward the marital partner (particularly if the partner has the infertility diagnosis or is more highly invested in parenthood). Whether a couple's experience of infertility involves actual pregnancy loss or the loss of the child they have dreamt of having, the psychological experience of infertility is as a narcissistic injury and a *symbolic* loss of self (Leon, 1990).

For most people, infertility is a psychological crisis and trauma. Whether it turns out to be a short-term or long-term trauma for a couple, the psychological effects are usually the same. Infertility shakes the foundations of how people feel about themselves as men and women, how they feel about their self worth, and their body. Infertility disrupts their faith in a benevolent, predictable, and meaningful world. It means grieving the losses of life goals, status, prestige, self-confidence, and assumption of fertility, loss of health, loss of pregnancies, or babies that could or should have been. It may also involve mourning relationships that were altered, slipped away and were lost, or are forever changed because of infertility. For most infertile men and women, the list of losses attributable to infertility is far longer than they imagined.

Bereavement is fundamental to infertility. Most couples entering infertility clinics are normal, healthy adults—-not "patients." They are not expecting a "patient" experience or extensive medical interventions, but assistance with what they assume (or hope) is a minor problem. With a diagnosis and treatment plan, they are catapulted into the sobering world of reproductive medicine in which, over time, they learn more than they ever wanted or expected to know about a field of medicine many did not previously know even existed. This phenomenon has been described as "paradise lost," or the dawning awareness of the stark reality that complex medical treatment is a necessity if one wishes to become a parent.

Couples experiencing infertility often begin by grieving their lost "health" or "normalcy" and end by grieving a multitude of losses. The grief of infertility may be an intense blow at the very outset of treatment (e.g., azoospermia, hysterectomy due to cancer) or a gradual accumulation of losses over time (e.g., sexual spontaneity, friendships). Grieving typically involves the narcissistic injuries inflicted by the feelings of personal failure, isolation, guilt, shame, envy, rage, and self-blame common to infertility. Grief, guilt, and envy are often commingled as the infertile patient feels jealous of others with babies or who are pregnant and then feels ashamed and guilty about these feelings. This becomes another in the long list of losses from infertility: the not-me of the person's "recognizable self."

According to Erickson (1950), persons in adulthood are attempting to move from *identity versus role confusion* into the *generativity versus stagnation* stage of life. For infertile persons, remaining "stuck" and unable to proceed to the next developmental stages (i.e., generativity) feels like "being in limbo," remaining in an indeterminate, ambiguous state—being forced by circumstances to be self-absorbed with the self-involvement focusing on their infertility and reproductive goals. Because the longed-for child is "psychologically present but physically absent," the boundaries of their marital system are ambiguous (Burns, 1987).

Infertility represents the loss of a fantasy or hope of fulfilling an important fantasy, the loss of the future and past in the potential child or child that *should* be. The ambiguous boundaries of infertile couples are emotionally painful and can have longlasting effects for the infertile couples because over time the longed-for child becomes an idealized child who represents idealized portions of each spouse (Burns, 1987). On the other hand, the failure of the child to arrive may be perceived as caused by the negative characteristics (faults) of oneself or one's partner. Involuntary childlessness represents both a narcissistic loss and an ambiguous loss (the loss of the longed-for child who is psychologically present but physically absent).

A couple's ability to manage the experience of infertility in a healthy fashion is typically contingent on their individual and relationship health going into the experience, their coping mechanisms, and their ability to find avenues for acknowledging the loss, expressing their emotions, and managing the crisis. While infertility may be "resolved" by the achievement of parenthood, it leaves a legacy—often affecting the couple's adjustment to parenthood and, consequently, their children (Burns, 1990, 1999). The need to rework or reexperience parts of infertility is a bitter pill for most previously infertile individuals and couples, particularly if a prominent coping mechanism during infertility was "It will all be better when I have a baby. This pain will evaporate then."

APPROACHES TO TREATMENT

The tasks and journeys of therapy change over the course of the psychological changes of infertility and depend, to a large extent, on which point in their infertility treatment journey a person or couple seeks assistance. However, there are some generalities. The goals of therapy include healing the narcissistic wounds of infertility, restoring self-esteem, and bereavement therapy. Bereavement often includes the possible loss of a potential child, while later in the couple's treatment it may entail grieving the loss of a biological child (e.g., miscarriages; post-IVF "chemical" pregnancy).

Because infertility is such a multifaceted experience affecting health, reproduction, family, social dynamics, and other intrapsychic and interpersonal aspects of the infertile person's and couple's life, treatment modalities are typically not limited to a single approach. Therapeutic approaches that have been applied to infertility include psychodynamic therapy, cognitive-behavioral treatment, marriage and family therapy, group therapy, strategic/solution-focused brief therapy, psychopharmacological treatment, sex therapy, crisis intervention, and grief counseling (Applegarth, 1999).

Although not a great deal of research has been done on evidence-based medicine and the efficacy of a particular treatment modality, it is generally recognized that a variety of treatment modalities (individual, couple, family, support, and therapy groups) is the most effective approach. Additionally, most infertility counselors take an interactive approach (versus the approach of classical psychoanalysis) perhaps because many have experienced infertility themselves (Covington and Marosek, 1999) or because infertile patients elicit this sort of self–other relational interaction that is unique to the crisis of infertility. In the therapeutic relationship, infertility counselors often offer advice, education, consultation, support, and analysis; and they are more likely to be patient advocates with caregivers or health care providers than in more traditional psychotherapies (Burns and Covington, 1999).

What follows are case examples that illustrate the evolution of psychological changes for infertile couples over the course of infertility. These examples include cases that address male factor infertility; donor gametes; infertility complicated by concomitant physical illness; infertility complicated by preexisting mental health problems; and infertility with remarriage issues.

MALE FACTOR INFERTILITY

John and Sally had been trying to conceive for two years, had been diagnosed with male factor infertility, and had sought counseling because they had begun to experience sexual problems. John dominated the sessions with intellectual discussions of his diagnosis, his frustration that his identical twin brother did not have fertility problems, and his irritation with the couple's respective doctors. Sally sat quietly, seldom adding anything to the session and then only briefly when addressed directly. Although one could *feel* each partner's sadness and anger, John and Sally would not acknowledge their feelings even when confronted or encouraged.

During the third session, John was assigned the "homework" of finding some way to express his anger. At the next session he reported he had gone to the driving range and hit golf balls. After a pause, I said impulsively, "It's interesting to me that you went out to hit *balls*." John laughed and said, "I guess I really am angry with my balls." What followed was a flood of feelings that ended with tears. While John talked and wept, Sally held his hand. After John eventually fell silent, Sally said, very quietly, "You know, I have been playing a lot more golf lately myself." John and I stared at her in disbelief—not sure if we could be confident about what she had just acknowledged. Sally smiled at herself, but when neither John nor I laughed or smiled, she looked to John as if asking permission to continue. When he nodded, she allowed herself to talk about her feelings, which included how she felt she "should" protect John from her angry feelings and take the "blame" for their diagnosis with their family and friends. She did not want to burden him with her feelings and make him feel even worse.

Sally and John are an example of many of the typical responses to male factor infertility. While ordinarily wives are more likely to be distressed about infertility than their husbands are, this is typically not the case when infertility is owed to male factor. Infertile men are more likely to experience a sense of stigma, loss of potency, role failure, and diminished self-esteem (Nachtigall, Becker, and Wozny, 1992). John talked about the isolation of male factor infertility and of feeling incapable of talking to anyone, even his twin, about his infertility. He also talked about language that denigrates infertile men: "He's got no balls," "That takes brass balls," "That's a ball buster."

John, like most infertile men, felt guilt and lowered self-esteem. Like other infertile men, who are less likely to grieve appropriately, John had defended against his feelings (e.g., intellectualization and repression) (Newman and Houle, 1993). Infertile men often experience denial or apportion blame either to themselves or to their female partners in order to shift the burden through projection or to make the diagnosis more culturally acceptable (e.g., in Middle Eastern countries). Men also feel marginalized and isolated and are less likely than women to seek assistance (Zoldbrod and Covington, 1999). Finally, Sally and John interacted around the issue of male factor infertility as many couples do: the wife protecting her husband either by openly taking the blame or by passively letting others believe their infertility is owed to female factor.

The decision to be spontaneous or even provocative in therapy is one most therapists struggle with at some point. Both restraint and spontaneity can be either thoughtful or thoughtless—a fact of which I was keenly aware when considering my response to John's disclosure about hitting golf balls. The struggle with restraint and spontaneity is a central feature of the therapist's craft and one with which a therapist continually reconsiders past decisions and their sequelae. According to Mitchell (2000), this struggle helps the therapist expand and enrich the context in which current therapeutic choices are made while at the same time highlighting the bidirectional/interactive nature of psychotherapy. This is an example of the phenomenon that occurred early in my career as an infertility counselor and has been often reconsidered and reevaluated. When reconsidering this intervention, I recall feelings of apprehension as well as an awareness that John's statement was the most "feeling" comment he had made in therapy (thereby exemplifying the importance of what is *unsaid or unfelt* in therapy as much as the importance of what *is* said).

Sally, John, and I discussed my remark later in the session and later in our therapeutic relationship. It was a very blunt comment, and I wondered if they were offended or felt it was inappropriate.

However, they felt it was a very useful intervention that had broken the ice in a significant (and humorous) way. Although in some ways my response surprised me (primarily for its bluntness), in others, it did not. John had chosen to express his angry feelings by "hitting balls," which was significant because he had been unable to express his feelings directly. "Hitting balls" seemed very metaphorical and too important to let pass. There seemed no way around it but to point this out. Finally, the breakthrough allowed the couple to proceed with therapy in a much more productive manner, ultimately allowing them to achieve greater intimacy and to communicate in a much more honest fashion.

Sally's passivity and silence probably was an unconscious attempt to diminish her husband's feelings of impotence and enhance his feelings of power by allowing his intellectualization of their infertility problem. The therapeutic intervention (John's homework) was risky in that it could have increased his feelings of impotence. However, it actively took control of an obvious therapeutic impasse. It was a playful, yet powerful, comment that took an "interpretative whack" at the therapeutic impasse and effectively "struck" at John's intellectualization.

Levenson (1988) contends that patients present riddled with blindspots, inattentions, scotomata—all the result of their anxiety and need for a defense. Defenses can operate against a mosaic of dynamic implications so that what is avoided is not a single underlying dynamic but a "veritable swiss cheese of avoidances." This was the case for both John and Sally: each had a "veritable swiss cheese" of avoidances. Their avoidances made it very difficult to speak honestly to each other or move on to a greater emotional depth that was necessary for them to come to terms with their feelings about their infertility.

MENTAL HEALTH ISSUES AND MARITAL ISSUES

Jemma and Todd were seen for a pre-IVF preparation and education interview that is the protocol at their clinic. They reported positive marital functioning and excellent support from family, friends, their church, and their faith. However, with Todd's encouragement, Jemma disclosed that she felt she was "going crazy" and began to cry. She felt depressed, anxious, and that she was "reacting" to the fertility drugs. She had recently quit a prestigious job in her field to work part-time as a sales clerk in a gift shop in order to "reduce stress" and increase her chances of getting pregnant. She also reported panic attacks, needle phobia, and insomnia. Jemma readily agreed to return for counseling. She acknowledged that infertility had probably exacerbated preexisting undiagnosed or untreated mental health problems.

As IVF cycles failed and her ability to manage the infertility crisis diminished, Jemma further decompensated and her ability to cope deteriorated. As she vented her feelings of sadness, frustration, jealousy, grief, and distress, her husband, family, and medical caregivers became increasingly alarmed. Her parents and husband encouraged her to turn to prayer and arranged prayer vigils around the IVF "implantation" phase. However, when the IVF cycles failed, Jemma experienced a crisis of faith as well. Her parents' distress and her brothers' parenthood increased her feelings of isolation and abandonment. The relinquishment of her career and job without a resulting pregnancy increased her feelings that she had altered and adapted her life to accommodate infertility, all for nothing. She felt her world was whirling out of control and that all her efforts to gain control were ineffective.

Feeling alone and bereft, Jemma turned to her husband as her sole source of "real" support. However, as her distress mounted and her neediness increased, he pulled away—put off and overwhelmed by her distress. He *did* want to support her but also felt that her emotions left no room for *his* feelings. Furthermore, he felt he did not recognize his wife as she was now: the Jemma affected by infertility compared with the accomplished and capable woman whom he had married. His withdrawal increased Jemma's feelings of abandonment and further destabilized the marriage. Eventually Todd became so concerned about Jemma's emotional well-being that he demanded that the couple terminate treatment and pursue adoption. This decision proved a significant motivation for her in psychotherapy, and she was able to convince her husband to do "one more" IVF cycle during which she promised to remain "emotionally steady" no matter what the outcome. However, when she became pregnant with twins, all her anxieties became focused on the pregnancy and then the children. Jemma was very dismayed to discover that pregnancy and impending parenthood did not provide her with instant "evaporation" or "disappearance" of her worries and concerns or the legacy of infertility.

Jemma and Todd's marital issues arose primarily as a result of Jemma's demands and inability to control her emotions. Todd's withdrawal and self-protection was interpreted by Jemma as rejection and abandonment—feelings all too familiar to her from her family of origin. Infertility is a unique marital crisis that involves the loss of a part of self or identity fundamental to each partner. Through therapy, Jemma was able to hear her husband's feelings and alter her response to him and to infertility accordingly. Ultimately, that she was highly motivated to "stay steady" during the final IVF cycle demonstrated to herself and to her husband her ability to cope successfully with the painful feelings of infertility, thereby drawing them closer.

Although Jemma initially described her family as supportive, in fact, they did not really understand either the depth of her feelings or the medical treatments she was undergoing. Furthermore, both of her younger brothers' wives were pregnant, and the experience of pregnancies, births, and new babies triggered overwhelming sadness, jealously, anger, and distress in her. Jemma felt guilty and ashamed of these feelings, yet despite her best efforts, family gatherings were excruciating and not enjoyable as they "should be." Her feelings of guilt about her jealous feelings increased her feelings of conflicting loyalties to the various versions of herself as well as all the significant others in her life (Mitchell, 2000). When Jemma spoke to her parents, she was surprised to learn about *their* sadness and was particularly distressed when her father's only response was tears. Jemma's idealization of her father and her family system left her feeling bereft. Because she could not live up to her ideal image of herself, Jemma felt guilty and ashamed. Infertility made Jemma feel helpless, ugly, and impotent. In reality, the family that Jemma initially described as "supportive" proved to be far more complex and complicated than Jemma had originally been willing to acknowledge. Psychotherapy allowed Jemma's perception of her family to become more nuanced, textured, and honest.

This case was challenging for me as it mirrored, in many ways, my own experiences with infertility. I recalled having struggled with issues of loss of control, the existential meaning of infertility, and the feeling that I was "going crazy." I quit my job in hopes of "increasing my odds" of pregnancy, felt alienated from family members who were able to have children while I was not, and eventually had the issue of infertility affect my marriage. Years later, my husband told me he had not recognized the person I became during infertility and, although it was difficult for me to hear or admit, I myself had not recognized that person either.

Now, listening to Jemma and Todd, I found countertransference issues emerging and had difficulty staying in the session. I found myself recalling my own experience and had difficulty staying in the "here-and-now." Despite countertransference issues, I was very aware it had been 30 years since my own infertility, and what I had to offer this couple was stability and perspective. I could contain Jemma's strong affective state as she tried to bring stability back to her life. Another way to interpret our interaction was that Jemma's reaction to her infertility triggered my negative memories. My capacity to tolerate my own different self-states triggered stability in her, rather than shaming her or making her feel guilty. As stability occurred, Todd was able to react in a less blaming way and be more accessible. Thus, therapeutically helping her to contain her "craziness," helped her to become more stable. As is so often the case, one's personal memories and experiences can be helpful in stabilizing patients particularly if the therapist is able to remain fluid in time and recall different self-states. This was the case for Jemma and enabled her to tolerate more complex feelings and self-states.

HEALTH ISSUES AND INFERTILITY

David and Mimi met in college and married soon after graduation. Mimi was an attractive, petite, even tiny woman who worked in corporate marketing. In her early 20s, soon after the death of her mother, Mimi was diagnosed with a rare bone disease making pregnancy risky if not impossible. Throughout the couple's 15-year marriage, Mimi had wanted children but David had discouraged it because of her health problems. The couple presented at an infertility clinic asking for medical treatment to achieve a pregnancy but were referred for counseling because reports from the perinatologist and rheumatologist advised against pregnancy. Mimi found it impossible to understand or accept the fact that she could not carry a pregnancy and wept copiously during most therapy sessions.

David, who was a reserved and introspective man, came to each session and comforted his wife while she grieved and vented her feelings of frustration, injustice, and powerlessness. Eventually the couple confided that they had sexual intercourse only once or twice a year. Both partners agreed that this was David's choice. David stated that by not having sex with his wife he could insure she would not become pregnant and her health would not be endangered. He felt (accurately) that Mimi did not listen to him, her physicians, or anyone else and was willing to risk her life for a pregnancy if left to her own devices. Her inability to see the matter "sensibly" or discuss it "rationally" had led David to withdraw from physical and emotional intimacy altogether; instead he played video games and watched endless TV sporting events. "He's present but not present," she complained—an observation that appeared to be true.

When he finally talked about his feelings, David wept, stating he could not imagine living without his wife, and no baby or anyone else would be worth losing her. He had watched the vicissitudes of her illness and said, "Sometimes I think it is worse for the person who is watching than for the person who is sick—but that sounds unkind. I know it can't be." Additionally, he feared that, if the couple did become parents, Mimi's health would continue to decline and he would end up being the sole caregiver of her and a child, a burden that he felt was beyond him since he was an only child and responsible for his ailing mother.

This case is an excellent example of infertility compounding feelings of body betrayal, helplessness, and hopelessness. It is also exemplifies covert marital conflict and sexual dysfunction. Mimi and David were stuck in an unspoken, covert marital conflict. He had passively withdrawn into a silent world of his own, unilaterally winning a silent "victory" to maintain his wife's health. It was interesting to observe how David played out this same defense mechanism (being present but not present) in therapy. David was a perfect example of the "best way to understand someone is their relations with others, past and present" (Mitchell, 2000, p. 107). David's passive, yet firm, determination to protect his wife's health was a communication pattern neither partner found easy to examine. However, with the issues stated openly and clearly, it became easier for them to move forward toward greater intimacy (their sexual relationship improved) and resolution (together they made a plan to adopt).

This couple presented with a grieving style described as the "keening syndrome" (Burns and Covington, 1999). In it, the wife openly grieves the various losses of infertility and in doing so assumes the role of the primary mourner, bearing an unequal share of the emotional burden of infertility. While the wife mourns, the husband expresses his grief by remaining silent, engaging in solitary (or secret) grief, or becoming immersed in activity (or distraction) (Staudacher, 1991). The husband becomes a silent, "forgotten" mourner in the process of grieving infertility. David and Mimi (like Jemma and Todd) fit this pattern perfectly, particularly in the early sessions, when Mimi was unable to control her weeping and David sat quietly offering nonverbal comfort. As David was encouraged to discuss his feelings, he found emotional relief in expressing them, while Mimi found relief in sharing the emotional burden of infertility. Although some of David's feelings were painful and difficult for Mimi to hear and accept, they brought the couple closer and increased their emotional intimacy. Sexual intimacy improved, particularly once the couple had *openly* agreed that a pregnancy was not an alternative for them.

Mimi still had considerable work to do on health and body issues, but this would be an ongoing struggle for her. When she began therapy, she simply could not believe that pregnancy would jeopardize her health despite what she had been told by her various physicians. Her denial took its toll on her intrapsychically as well as interpersonally (e.g., in her marriage). Mimi's self-image took a double blow with the loss of health and reproduction at the same time. Responding with denial, she stated that "the risk was worth it to her" even though none of her caregivers or her husband believed she really understood what she was saying or meant it if she did. The loss of her mother at the time of her diagnosis helped entrench repression of powerful, threatening feelings of overwhelming grief that had become, with infertility, disorganizing emotional experiences. She believed that, by achieving the miracle of pregnancy, she could bring back her mother, the mother who is both present and absent. Mimi looked to parenthood to replace these various losses, bolster her self-esteem and place her back into the world of "normalcy" and health.

Over the course of my work with this couple, I was diagnosed with a serious illness. This experience broadened my therapeutic perspective of Mimi's experience while at the same time causing the eruption of all sorts of countertransference issues. I developed a greater empathy for the challenges of her illness and its impact on her life; how and why denial was an effective coping (defense) mechanism; and the difficulties of redirecting one's life when health has prevented one from going in the direction one had originally planned. Mimi clung to a definition of herself as normal (e.g., able to carry a pregnancy) and did not want to be identified "as her illness." Her denial helped her maintain a sense of herself as normal and "just like everyone else" and not see herself as "only an illness." However, denial had also prevented her from redirecting her life on the basis of limits imposed by her illness. Initially, I was reluctant to share my personal experience with illness, but this became inevitable when I was required to reduce my work schedule and explain why to Mimi and John. My explanation was instrumental for Mimi as we discussed how difficult it is to "adjust" and "realign" one's life in the face of health problems, particularly if one appears perfectly healthy. While I had very ambivalent feelings about sharing this personal issue, it proved to be immensely helpful for Mimi and David; and, by helping them, it helped me too.

INFERTILITY AND PRIOR SEXUAL TRAUMA

Dylan and Peggy met when Peggy was traveling in Dylan's native Ireland and they later married there. They had never used birth control during their seven-year marriage. They had undergone ovulation induction at Peggy's ob/gyn clinic but had never conceived. They were referred to an infertility clinic where a physician ordered a semen analysis, which had never been done previously. However, Dylan objected to this testing and the couple chose to do donor insemination instead. During the donor gamete preparation and educational interview, Dylan explained that he was not opposed to the semen analysis on religious grounds but was uncomfortable with the "process" of semen collection. Peggy did not understand her husband's objections but passively and unquestioningly accepted them, accurately recognizing his emotional distress. With some gentle encouragement, Dylan finally shared that, while growing up, he had attended Roman Catholic boys' schools in Ireland where he had suffered significant sexual abuse over several years. Peggy was unaware of this history of sexual trauma and wept while her husband talked about it for the first time. He felt relieved that his experiences had not "ruined" or "tarnished" his marriage but feared he would be retraumatized if he "went down that road again" by masturbating for the semen analysis.

Dylan rejected the idea of further counseling but was grateful that his wife now knew what he had gone through. Given this new information, Peggy now felt she wanted to table the decision to pursue donor insemination, and Dylan agreed. The couple was given suggestions for making the collection process more acceptable and not traumatizing for Dylan, including collection at home with special condoms. Dylan was found to have a slightly low sperm count, and the couple underwent a husband insemination/ovulation induction cycle by collecting in the manner recommended. They became pregnant during their first treatment cycle and did not return for psychotherapy. However, on a visit to the clinic to show off their baby son, Dylan stopped me in the clinic hallway to thank me for "making him talk about that topic." Dylan offered that, if had he not been encouraged to talk about it, they would not have "this little bugger."

This case well illustrates male factor infertility as well as guilt issues related to sexuality. As stated earlier, research indicates that women seem to experience infertility with greater distress then men do unless it is male factor infertility diagnosis. However, for Dylan this was not truly a diagnosis of infertility or even male factor. This couple had not even been systematically evaluated for infertility although they had undergone considerable treatment. As a result, they were making their reproductive decisions on the basis of Dylan's previous sexual abuse, although this was unknown to his wife or caregivers. Dylan had not discussed his painful past and took the blame for the abuse onto himself. Having learned to internalize the negative with abuse, he did the same with reproduction. He was willing to proceed with donor insemination (a form of self-deprivation and self-punishment) rather than confess to his caregivers or wife his reasons for not wanting to proceed with a semen analysis. He remained isolated, ashamed, and grieving until faced with very significant reproductive decisions.

When Dylan was a youngster, his parents divorced and his mother relocated to the United States while his father remarried and lived in Ireland. Dylan and his brothers were sent "away to school." Dylan, like many abused children, had no comfort, no one who modeled healthy ways of coping or offered solace if he verbalized what had happened (McWilliams, 1999). Having learned to keep silent about his abuse, Dylan did not share the experience of abuse in the emotionally intimate relationship of marriage even though it was a very close one. He felt that he needed to protect his wife from the abuse or she or their relationship would be "spoiled" by the abuse in the same way that he felt he had been. The instant (but operationally different) comfort and support from both the therapist and his wife encouraged Dylan to rework his view of this experience. And although he refused a referral for other therapeutic interventions, I speculate that his improved communication with his wife was a significant intervention as was the achievement of parenthood—a son whom "he was going to treat differently."

Davies and Frawley (1994) speculate that abuse involves a triad: the abuser, the abused, and the "helpless" other who does not "know" about the abuse, does not pay attention to it, but allows the abuse to continue. Dylan's parents were, in many ways, the helpless others. Although they did not know about the abuse, they certainly knew that Dylan was not happy at the boarding schools he attended. Dylan blamed them for going about their own lives without considering their children. His parents felt that if the school fees were paid they had done their duty. His father was an alcoholic (albeit functional) who continued to live in Ireland, yet rarely visited his son, while his mother had remarried and started over with a new family.

In adulthood, Dylan maintained a very distant relationship with both parents. He described his anger and resentment toward his parents; the Roman Catholic clergy who had abused him; and the Roman Catholic Church in general. In addition, he described his fears about how his wife and marriage would be affected by this information: would Peggy think him a homosexual? Peggy felt this was a ridiculous fear but said so in a respectful way, careful not to blurt out her first response, which she shared later: "How could you think such a thing?"

Often, the therapist takes the role of authority in treatment by taking control of the situation through gentle and careful inquiry—in this case about Dylan's and Peggy's lack of semen analysis. By my doing so, Peggy was not allowed to remain in the position of the helpless other—she could and would now share the experience (and burden of it) with Dylan. In addition to taking control, this was an example of modeling helpful authority—something Dylan very much needed. This couple could have fallen into the pitfalls of infertility treatment and medical authority figures that would have left Dylan (and perhaps Peggy) feeling again abused. Instead, this was an example of an authority that helped, cared when he "confessed" his sin, and illuminated forgiveness (for himself) and his wife's unquestioning forgiveness.

This case stands out in my memory because, as so often happens in a session or with a case, there was a feeling during the session that "something does not add up here." The couple that sat before me was attractive, intelligent, well groomed, and clearly devoted to one another. Often a therapist's sixth sense is awareness that there is more to the story but ignorance of what it is exactly. Although this couple presented for educational and preparation counseling for donor insemination (as required by their clinic), there was something about them and their brief infertility history that did not make sense. Why had they not had a semen analysis at their previous clinic? Why would they be willing to proceed with donor insemination (the relinquishment of biological parenthood for Dylan) without even minimal investigation? Clearly

Dylan had strong feelings or Peggy would not have been so compliant as she confessed her longing for a child that was "part of both of us." One always wonders whether to pay attention to these intuitions and, if so, how to go about investigating them so that individuals and couples do not feel traumatized or invaded. Being respectful, but gently probing, is helpful, but not always as gratifying as this case.

AGE AND REMARRIAGE ISSUES

Connie was a 41-year-old high school teacher who had been married to her husband, Jack, 52 years old, for 12 years. It was the first marriage for Connie and the second for Jack, who was divorced when his only son was a year old. Jack shared custody of his son, Liam, age 14, although now Liam spent more time with his father and stepmother by his choice. Connie and Jack had been trying to conceive for most of their marriage, but the cause of infertility was unknown and their efforts had been unsuccessful. Now, at age 41, Connie agreed with her physicians that age was becoming a major factor for both her and her husband. Early in the couple's marriage she had been confident and determined about having a child; her husband agreed only because it was what she wanted. Now she was ambivalent while her husband had become openly opposed to more children. He looked forward to the time when Liam would go to college and they could travel and enjoy the benefits of an empty nest.

Connie had initially hoped to create a bond with her stepson by providing him a stepsibling. Now, with Liam 14 years old and clearly passing through the separation and individuation stage of his life, cementing an attachment to an infant sibling was less likely to happen. All this brought to the surface Connie's ambivalent feelings about her role as stepmother and her feelings about motherhood in general. Liam's mother saw him as her primary source of emotional support and companionship and had never set any rules or boundaries. He was more her peer than a son. By contrast, his father and stepmother set clear parental boundaries and limits. Although Liam rebelled against the rules of the house, he chose to spend more and more of his time with Connie and Jack, but he often fought with or openly rebelled against Connie. As a result, Connie viewed stepparenting as unrewarding and longed for a "child of my own" who would provide her with more rewarding experiences of parenting and motherhood.

This case illustrates the unique issues of age and remarriage as they apply to infertility. Many infertility patients do not start treatment in the older range of their reproductive lives but reach it over the course of their treatment. As the months and years of treatment pass, they suddenly realize that their chances of conceiving have considerably diminished because of their age, and pregnancy now involves a wide array of previously unforeseen risks and complications (i.e., increased risk of miscarriage and birth defects). And, while pregnancy is more complicated and complex, so is parenthood. Older first-time parenthood can mean postponing retirement, caring for an infirm spouse and young children simultaneously, and different financial burdens as well as social issues, such as being mistaken as a grandparent instead of a parent.

As Connie began to investigate her feelings about discontinuing medical treatment, the diminishing odds of success at her age, and her husband's feelings about second parenthood, she was able to differentiate the difference between then and now. She could see that where she had begun was not where she was now and that she had to evaluate her thoughts and feelings according to the current situation, not what could have been or should have been. She could then grieve the child she had assumed she would have and all the additional losses of not having that child.

Connie began to deal with the issues all mothers must address: reviewing how she was mothered. Her father died when she was a toddler, and her mother was a neglectful, emotionally absent, alcoholic parent. Connie had had to "mother myself as well as my younger siblings." She felt equally angry with her stepson (particularly his adolescent rebellions with her) and his mother, of whom she was critical. Connie's rage was displacement of the anger she felt toward her father, whose death had left her feeling abandoned. In addition, it represented her feelings of jealousy toward the "bad mothers" (who have the ability to reproduce) and good mothers (like Connie, who as the ideal good mother, cannot reproduce).

Connie's drive to be a mother was based in her desire to recreate her family while creating an ideal family of her own in which she could "do it over and get it right." She did not consider stepparenthood to be "real mothering" or parenthood and instead dreamed of having her own "ideal child" for whom she would be the ideal mother. In this fantasy, she did not address the issues of attachment, object constancy, internalization of other, and separation-individuation central to actual mothering. Like many stepparents or simply infertile women, she thought she could and would do this when she became a mother—not in her role as stepmother. However, in reality, Connie was operating as a mother in Liam's life: providing him with a more nourishing and healthy relationship than his actual mother did, as represented by his rebellious interactions with her. Liam was more comfortable with their interactions because of the parental boundaries that were firm but permeable and the fact that Connie did not use him for emotional support as his mother did.

As Connie began to investigate her feelings about motherhood and her own mother, she found that her anger, hurt, and rage at her mother was at a depth she had never imagined. "I cannot be in the same room with her for more than a half hour without a fight breaking out." Connie's facing her feelings about her mother and her reasons for them relieved her of considerable pain and helped her move on from infertility and invest to a greater degree in her role as stepmother. Connie considered how she had played an important role as Liam's mother in his life since he was three years old by attending school conferences, celebrations, and sharing vacations. She imagined how the future would remain the same—graduations, his wedding, and grandchildren.

Psychotherapy with Connie included facilitation of bereavement; exploring issues of motherhood and stepparenting; exploring family-of-origin issues; and exploring her ego defenses and relational expectations, particularly as they related to her desire for another child and her role as stepmother. With Connie's work on the issue of motherhood, she was able to let go of her desire and need to pursue infertility treatment. She and her husband began making plans for before and after Liam went to college. Her relationship with Liam improved. His schoolwork and behavior improved, and they developed a shared hobby: chess tournaments to which they traveled together throughout the country. Her relationship with her mother did not improve except that Connie was able to place acceptable boundaries on it (e.g., no telephone calls after the cocktail hour). An unexpected side effect was that these boundaries provided a model for Liam for handling his own mother.

This case involved a number of countertransference issues, particularly those related to pregnancy and parenthood in older couples. Connie was only 29 and not an older primagravidum when she began trying to conceive 12 years ago, nor was her husband "too old." But now, at 41, her reproductive age was quite different and involved many risks that couples do not consider: decreased fertility in both men and women; increased risk of miscarriage; increased risk of pregnancy-related problems for the mother (e.g., hypertension, gestational diabetes); and increased risk of birth defects in the infant. Very frequently, couples are not only not aware of these age-related risks, they do not want to hear about them. This reluctance can trigger countertransference issues, particularly those relating to the quest for the perfect baby while denying the potential risks.

A unique countertransference issue in this case was Connie's narrow definition of motherhood. Like so many women, Connie defined motherhood in reproductive terms, a definition that is always a source of sadness for me. It is my belief that children as well as adults can gain so much from defining these roles in far broader terms. However, I was able to help Connie see how her experiences as a mother with Liam were the same as my own experience as a mother or that of any mother and, as such, a significant part of his attachment to her.

CONCLUSION

Paul Tillich (1958), a Protestant theologian, stated that "grace is accepting the unacceptable" (p. 127). For me, adjustment to infertility is accepting infertility as unacceptable—internalizing the unacceptable nature of infertility. Infertility will never be acceptable in the lives of the men and women who experience it. It will never be an experience that they look back on with positive and pleasant feelings or memories, even if they eventually become parents along the way. Infertility will always be *unacceptable* because what it involves and entails is in contrast to how they thought they would become parents. Infertility is, by definition, an interruption of normal biological process and life stages. It is an anathema to what they felt and believed in and entailed so much that was abhorrent—as such, infertility can never be acceptable. It will always be unacceptable. The goal of therapy, then, is being able to live comfortably with *accepting the unacceptable*.

This acceptance begins when the losses of infertility become increasingly integrated into the individual's and the couple's life and no longer is their life focus. The couple are able to expand their attention, energy, and emotions to a broader view, perhaps considering adoption or a childless life. They are able to include others in their world, perhaps to mourn with them and prevent infertility from negatively affecting their relationships and lives. This process may be one in which the couple has found their inner resources or been helped to become aware of them, or it may be that life's events have drawn the couple away from the trauma and grief of infertility and down new avenues.

Fundamental to the recovery from infertility (or any trauma) is finding some way to give the experience meaning. Viktor Frankl (1946), a psychiatrist who survived World War II concentration camp internment, investigated the existential question: What is suffering and why am I experiencing it? Although the pain of involuntary childlessness is not comparable to concentration camp imprisonment, the pain and suffering it involves is comparable to major illness and life crises and, consequently, triggers the same existential questions. To recover from the infertility experience, men and women must, at least over time if not in the moment, give their suffering and the experience of infertility some meaning. Infertility cannot remain a meaningless experience in their lives. It must be defined in some way: perhaps as an experience from which they learned about themselves as a couple and how to cope with trauma or how they grew as individuals. By giving the experience meaning, the individual and couple become aware of their own resources and their resiliency—their ability to weather any storm no matter how tempestuous.

Working with infertile patients is challenging because their grief becomes our own, their existential questions activate our own existential issues, their trauma triggers our own grief experiences. While it is important for therapists to maintain appropriate boundaries, they must also remain genuine and available during these painful struggles. They must maintain the delicate balance between disclosure and nondisclosure. They most provide therapeutic assistance while not depleting their own internal resources. Doing so can be a form of modeling healthy coping and management of feelings. The therapeutic goal for infertile persons and couples is to reach the resolution stage of infertility with their relationships intact, emotionally healthy, and having matured and grown stronger as a result of managing the crisis with courage and wisdom. Recently a patient asked (as many have over the years) if I had experienced infertility. When I answered only that I had, but many years ago, she said, "I don't want to know anything more than that. Just that you have is all I need to know." It occurred to me that that is what I would have liked to have heard when I was undergoing treatment. It would have made it easier and been very comforting. Now I was pleased that my journey could provide her the lifeline she needed.

REFERENCES

Applegarth, L. D. (1999), Individual counseling and psychotherapy. In: *Infertility Counseling: A Comprehensive Handbook for Clinicians*, ed. L. H. Burns & S. N. Covington. New York: Parthenon, pp. 85–101.

Burns, L. H. (1987), Infertility as boundary ambiguity: One theoretical perspective. *Family Process*, 26:359–372.

———— (1990), An exploratory study of perceptions of parenting after infertility. *Family Systems Med.*, 8:177–189.

———— & Covington, S. N., eds. (1999a), *Infertility Counseling: A Comprehensive Handbook for Clinicians*, ed. L. H. Burns & S. N. Covington. New York: Parthenon.

———— & ———— (1999b), Psychology of infertility. In: *Infertility Counseling:*

A Comprehensive Handbook for Clinicians, ed. L. H. Burns & S. N. Covington. New York: Parthenon, pp. 3–25.

Covington, S. N. (1999), Integrating infertility counseling into clinical practice. In: *Infertility Counseling: A Comprehensive Handbook for Clinicians*, ed. L. Burns & S. N. Covington. New York: Parthenon, pp. 475–490.

———— & Marosek, K. (1999), Personal infertility experience among nurses and mental health professionals working in reproductive medicine. Presented at meeting of American Society for Reproductive Medicine, September, Toronto.

Davies, J. M. & Frawley, M. G. (1994), *Treating the Adult Survivor of Childhood Sexual Abuse: A Psychoanalytic Perspective*. New York: Basic Books.

Erickson, E. (1950), *Childhood and Society*. New York: Norton Press.

Frankl, V. (1946), *Man's Search for Meaning*. New York: Washington Square Press.

Keye, W. R. (1999), Medical aspects of infertility for the counselor. In: *Infertility Counseling: A Comprehensive Handbook for Clinicians*, ed. L. H. Burns & S. N. Covington. New York: Parthenon, pp. 27–46.

Leon, I. (1990), *When a Baby Dies: Psychotherapy for Pregnancy and Newborn Loss*. New Haven, CT: Yale University Press.

Levenson, E. (1988), The pursuit of the particular. *Contemp. Psychoanal.*, 24:1–16.

McWilliams, N. (1999), *Psychoanalytic Case Formation*. New York: Guilford Press.

Mitchell, S. (2000), *Relationality: From Attachment to Intersubjectivity*. Hillsdale, NJ: The Analytic Press.

Nactigall, R. D., Beckers, G. & Wozny, M. (1992), The effects of gender-specific diagnosis on men's and women's response to infertility. *Fertility & Sterility*, 57:113–121.

Newman, C. R. & Houle, M. (1993), Gender differences in psychological responses to infertility treatment. In: *Psychological Issues in Infertility, Infertility and Reproductive Medicine Clinics of North America*, ed. D. A. Greenfeld. Philadelphia, PA: Saunders, pp. 545–558.

Staudacher, C. (1991), *Men and Grief*. Oakland, CA: New Harbinger.

Tillich, P. (1958), *Dynamics of Faith*. New York: Harper & Row, 2001.

Zoldbrod, A. P. & Covington, S. N. (1999), Recipient counseling for donor insemination. In: *Infertility Counseling: A Comprehensive Handbook for Clinicians*, ed. L. H. Burns & S. N. Covington. New York: Parthenon, pp. 325–344.

Part II

From the Therapist's Side

2

THERAPIST ANXIETY ABOUT
MOTIVATION FOR PARENTHOOD

Laura Josephs

Like many psychologists who focus on reproductive psychology, I became professionally involved with the world of infertility after I was personally (and painfully) drawn into this world. Though I managed to achieve a successful resolution of my infertility, I have not forgotten the raw feelings that accompanied being infertile: the deep disappointment, the anger, the acute sense of injustice. The fear that your sister, your sister-in-law, your best friend—in my case, my younger cousin—is going to turn up pregnant at Thanksgiving. The internal conflict around whether to skip someone's baby shower and feel guilty and excluded, or to go and feel wounded and inferior—and still excluded. I will not forget, either, the raw bodily experiences—being poked and prodded with various sharp implements in the effort to get pregnant; bloating from the medications; checking for blood in underwear or on toilet paper and, too often, finding it.

Now, as a psychologist working with infertile patients, I know that the person sitting in the room with me is probably not the person she was a year ago, not the person she was two years ago or at whatever point she began to try, with great hopes, to have a child. She is almost certainly sadder, angrier. She is likely less optimistic, more bitter. She is, probably not as "nice" as she used to be. Her psyche has been rubbed raw, as though a layer of defense has been peeled off.

EVALUATING MOTIVATION FOR PARENTHOOD

On one hand, I am a psychologist who consults in the area of reproductive medicine and who participates with an interdisciplinary team at a reproductive medicine program. Therefore, I am a representative of psychology in the world of reproductive medicine. On the other hand, I am a particular person. I have myself been affected by infertility. I remember how it felt to be denied the thing I wanted most, the only thing that seemed to matter. I remember how infertility can twist the psyche.

Perhaps my own experience, and not some rational, agreed-upon code of ethical principles, ends up being why, to this point, I have never put myself in the position of absolutely stopping someone from having a child. If an infertile patient is presenting with serious psychological difficulties, I tend to look at the ongoing narcissistic injury (that is, the infertility) that has undoubtedly exacerbated her preexisting difficulties. And I probably give patients plenty of leeway in motivation for parenthood. It is easy enough to dismiss patients' intense desires for a baby as springing from narcissistic strivings—a wish to be a success at reproducing and a wish to obtain a reflection of oneself, or a perfected version of oneself.

Within the world of infertility, the narcissistic aspects of the longing for a child become highly visible. Most of us, it turns out, are willing to go to pretty strenuous lengths—undergoing a myriad of invasive procedures—in order to have a child who is biologically and genetically related to us. Patients choosing a sperm donor look for men who are tall and handsome. And donor egg patients do not say things like, "I don't care what she [the donor] looks like." But if we all wanted children for the pure and noble reason of contributing to the next generation (rather than to reproduce ourselves, or some idealized version thereof), we would adopt an abandoned child at the first sign of reproductive failure, and fertility clinics would go out of business. And, when I found myself an infertility patient, was I any more noble than anybody else? I desperately wanted my own biological child, wanted to be a "success" at reproducing. Had I required egg donation, I am sure I would have wanted my donor to be reasonably attractive, not to mention very intelligent.

Thus, I have probably more or less accepted people's desire for a child at face value and have tended to interpret the quest to have a child as more or less a person's right, regardless of the subtle psychological motivations that fuel this desire. At the same time, I have had occasion to recommend the delay of childbearing—to patients themselves and, when I have served as a psychological consultant, to physicians providing assisted reproductive treatment. Perhaps to recommend delay is to empathize with the patient's basic motivation to have a child, while identifying the roadblocks to adequate parenting and, ideally, helping the patient to overcome these roadblocks. Here I will try to describe some of my internal struggles in working with people of questionable motivation for and readiness for parenthood, to describe some of the psychological and ethical principles that have informed my thinking and to discuss some of the decisions I have made or helped to make along the way.

Let me start with an extreme case. A 30-year-old woman, Mrs. C, was referred for psychological consultation by her reproductive endocrinologist (RE). Mrs. C authorized me to communicate with her reproductive endocrinologist concerning Mrs. C's evaluation and treatment. During the course of physical examination, the RE had discovered an unusual pattern of burns on the patient's abdomen, and the patient eventually told him that her husband had burned her, deliberately, with cigarettes.

Fortunately, unlike many victims of domestic violence, this patient was nearly emotionally ready to acknowledge the nature of her relationship with her partner and was willing to leave her abuser. They had been together for seven years, with a horrific picture of escalating sadistic abuse. In the consultation, it became clear that Mrs. C had convinced herself that becoming pregnant and having a child would stop the abuse and heal her violent marriage. At the same time, she realized that this was an unrealistic, desperate hope. Meanwhile, her self-esteem, low enough as a result of earlier life experiences when she entered into the relationship with her husband, was now—after years of verbal and physical abuse—abysmal, and infertility was making her feel herself to be "not a woman at all." Not surprisingly, she interpreted her inability to have a child as the ultimate sign of her essential undeservingness, as did her husband (who, of course, held her completely responsible for the infertility). In addition, feeling deeply unloved, Mrs. C longed for a baby to cherish and to hold.

My work with Mrs. C began with "denormalizing" the violence that had, in fact, become a "normal" part of her everyday existence and helping her to hold on to the frightening reality that she was living with someone who could easily kill her. To build her sense of self, I focused on helping her to stick consistently with a view of herself as undeserving of abuse and a recognition that her husband was a violent and pathological person who deserved to be imprisoned for his actions against her.

Neither the reproductive endocrinologist nor I needed to "stop" Mrs. C from pursuing infertility treatment. Despite an initial veneer of defensive denial, once the abuse was exposed to the light of day, Mrs. C herself knew that having a child in a situation where her life was literally in danger was completely untenable. At the same time, I was able to empathize with her *wish* for a child and with the pain of infertility. It was a relief to her when I told her that for women in stable life situations with loving partners, infertility was enough to decimate their self-esteem. On a practical level, I helped Mrs. C to obtain assistance from a victims' services organization. Mrs. C did not feel emotionally prepared to deal with calling the police, pressing charges, seeking an order of protection against her abusive husband, and so forth. She feared that her husband, once at liberty, would stalk and kill her. She was initially resistant to the idea of going to a shelter for battered women, in part, because she felt it was not fair (yet another unfairness) that she should be the one to lose her home and possessions. I was able to empathize with this sense of injustice but, of course, continued to confront her with the painful reality of her current choices.

Several months after our consultations began, I was thrilled to get a call from Mrs. C's sister, who told me that Mrs. C had asked her to call and tell me that Mrs. C had made it to a women's shelter and was safe.

Mrs. C's story is only partly one about infertility. To the degree that it is a story about infertility and about questionable parenthood, Mrs. C turned out to be easy to convince that her violent home was no place into which to bring a baby. But what if, instead, she had insisted on access to infertility treatment? I know that I would have recommended against this decision, and I am sure that her fertility doctor would have declined to provide treatment, because of his belief that providing treatment in this situation would have been, simply, wrong. Similarly, for most RE's who have been made aware that a given patient is being abused by her partner or is, herself, a serious alcohol or drug abuser, the physician would usually choose to withhold reproductive treatment until the abuse problem was resolved. Has any case like this ever gone to court—a case where extreme psychosocial circumstances meant the likelihood of a compromised pregnancy or a child's being born into a situation with a high potential for abuse? Technically perhaps a lawyer could make the point that everyone has the right of access to reproductive technology, and that the provider's responsibility is to make sure any resulting child receives proper protection from abuse or neglect. But, if ethics means doing what is right, can anyone fault the reproductive physician for declining to treat someone who is actively involved in an abusive existence? In real life, there surely are infertile patients who, unlike Mrs. C, persist in wanting to bring children into life situations that are incompatible with reasonable parenting. I believe that these patients end up seeking not a legal solution but a highly practical one: they simply go to a practitioner from whom they keep their problems secret, their private lives private.

In this free country, infertile persons end up with almost as much reproductive freedom as fertile people, for keeping one's private life private is usually easy enough. This is because no center for reproductive medicine is going to start doing background checks on its patients or interviewing these patients' neighbors about their daily habits. Because of the value society places on the basic right to reproduce and the reluctance of society to restrict this right, patients can readily conceal from practitioners even severe life problems. As a consultant in a hospital-based donor egg program, over the years I have assessed hundreds of couples seeking oocyte donation to have a child. Virtually all have denied current alcohol or substance abuse. Statistically, can that really represent an accurate picture? A certain percentage of these patients have to be hiding a substance problem from me, from themselves. All have denied domestic violence.

The donor egg program where I consult requires a psychological assessment for one to be placed on the waiting list for donation. When patients come to see me for this initial assessment, they present themselves very differently than do patients who come to see me for therapy. Part of the difference, of course, is that the latter group of patients have identified themselves as having a problem. But the other part of the difference is that the patients coming for donor egg consultation are looking to "present well," that is, to demonstrate a preponderance of socially desirable traits in themselves and in their relationship.

If presenting well, or "faking good," if you will, is what is striven for in a donor egg recipient consultation, a certain kind of significance is lent to that small percentage of patients who reveal, verbally or behaviorally, notable psychopathology during such consultations. I do not mean here the acknowledgment of hesitations, even strong reservations, about the use of donor gametes to conceive a child. I assume that gamete donation is never a first choice and that the prospective use of donor gametes means confronting the loss of the ability to use one's own genetic material to create a child. Notably, I also do not mean here simply the existence of psychopathology; in fact, a number of patients who were substance abusers in recovery, and at least one woman with a diagnosis of schizophrenia, have successfully come through the donor egg program.

But, a person showing significant unacknowledged pathology, or a couple revealing serious marital dysfunction during the one-hour clinical interview that is a requirement for participation in the egg donation program, has, I believe, quite a bit more meaning, for instance, than a couple seeking marital therapy and getting into a screaming match in their first session. The latter couple is, perhaps, getting into the issues that have brought them into treatment. What is the first couple communicating? They have come to present themselves as candidates for reproductive assistance. Instead they have ended up showing that their home life is likely highly problematic, that they are not accepting of gamete donation, or both.

When individuals or couples cannot "keep it together" during psychological evaluations for egg donation, I feel that these situations represent a "cry for help" to which I need to respond. Perhaps they started off with some psychological fragility, and years of negative IVF cycles or pregnancy losses have completely worn away at their psychological defenses. In these consultations, I have, on a number of occasions over the years, recommended that one or both members of a couple pursue psychotherapy. Often, these patients have agreed to this recommendation and have returned for a donor egg cycle some months later, when they have reached the top of the program's waiting list. But for some couples, a therapeutic confrontation and a recommendation for outside psychological treatment means that they will either not seek reproductive treatment or will, possibly, seek it elsewhere.

Mr. and Mrs. G, a childless couple in their early 40s, were referred for egg donation after years of failed IVF cycles and recent findings of poor ovarian reserve for Mrs. G. As part of the egg donation protocol at the hospital, they attended a psychological assessment session with me. We started off by discussing, briefly, their fertility treatment, but the consultation soon became an opportunity for Mrs. G to berate her husband for his unwillingness, years before, to begin trying to have a child with her. Mr. G acknowledged that he had delayed their attempts at child bearing for some months, perhaps a year, and appeared to be trying to empathize with his wife's feelings, but Mrs. G was relentless. Her harsh and pointed criticisms of her husband began with the issue of their infertility but soon branched out into a detailed description of a recent marital blowup and its aftermath, when Mrs. G left the house to go live with a friend for several weeks. She was furious at her husband because he had, apparently, passively waited for her to come home rather than pursuing her, as she had wished him to do. Mrs. G, out of control, screamed loudly at Mr. G and jabbed her finger in his face through much of her verbally abusive tirade.

Countertransferentially, during this consultation I found myself completely understanding why Mrs. G's husband had not made great efforts to contact her. In fact, I was thinking that he would have been much better off if he had decided to move during this time or at least to change the locks, along with his phone number! I also could not help thinking of their yet-to-be-conceived child. I imagined the child, at age one, spilling a cup of milk and of Mrs. G deciding that the child was deliberately trying to thwart her; or the child, at age three, not giving Mrs. G the response she desired and thereby becoming a target of her massive rage. My impression was that Mrs. G was a woman with borderline personality disorder, a likely "rage-aholic" who was ill equipped for parenthood. No doubt, apropos of my earlier comments regarding the stress of infertility, Mrs. G's psychological problems had worsened during years of failed attempts at conceiving a child. I was certain, however, that a pregnancy (in this case, a donor egg pregnancy) would not magically resolve her very serious problems. I confronted the couple with my assessment of them as having extremely serious marital difficulties and of Mrs. G as having very clear problems with her temper. Perhaps some, even many, of her grievances were legitimate in terms of content; it was clear, though, that the process whereby she conveyed her anger was highly dysfunctional.

Interestingly, Mrs. G did not appear to be highly defensive about my conclusions, even when I made it clear that I would recommend that donor egg treatment proceed only if they made a commitment to and seriously pursued some combination of marital and individual therapy with an outside therapist (or therapists). Both Mr. and Mrs. G stated that they would pursue outside therapy and that, in fact, they both believed that they should be in treatment. At the same time, Mrs. G noted that it was dealing with her husband that really "drove [her] crazy" and that it was he who required the lion's share of help.

Unsurprisingly the donor egg program never heard from Mr. and Mrs. G again. I am realistic enough to believe it unlikely that they sought psychological treatment and healed their troubled marriage. Did they split up, which seemed like a distinct possibility? Or did they just tell themselves that they were having a bad day when they came to see me and decide to seek donor egg treatment elsewhere, only this time they would make sure to be on good behavior if and when they met with the program psychologist?

For me, the G's in their consultation were basically telling me, "We're not ready to go forward with this." Was it the dynamic of this marriage that was causing Mrs. G to lose it, as she herself claimed? Was it the years of infertility that pushed her over the edge? Was she unable to accept the medical reality that donor egg was the only way for her to give birth to a child? Or was Mrs. G's behavior reflective of a longstanding pattern? Of course, I never had the opportunity to find out.

Had I been consulting with them in a different clinical context, both my intervention and the situation's outcome would have been different. I was meeting with the G's for assessment as part of their presentation as candidates for gamete donation, and I had their authorization to share the clinical information gleaned from this meeting with the egg donation program. In this model, the serious psychological problem they presented is akin to a medical problem, such as diabetes, which would need to be addressed and stabilized prior to their initiating fertility treatment. Had the G's instead been seeking private therapeutic help for their psychological problems, the nature of the consultation would have been different and I would have found myself in a different role.

In fact, I have met with more than one patient (though not many) over the years to whom I have said, "You shouldn't have a child now." Had I met with the G's in a private therapeutic context, that would be what I would say, and all I could say. Suppose they had been consulting with me privately for severe marital problems, or suppose Mrs. G had been meeting with me individually for her temper problem. I would have quickly confronted them, or her, with the folly of setting out to bring a child into their home before their troubled home life was better resolved. A psychologist in the role of evaluator can set a limit (i.e., tell individuals or couples that they need to resolve a serious psychological or substance abuse problem prior to infertility treatment), and this intervention can serve a useful function in breaking through a patient's denial about a disabling difficulty. But, ironically, when the psychologist as evaluator serves this limit-setting function, my experience is that he or she is rarely called on by the patient to help him or her follow through with the problem's resolution. It is when the mental health professional is not in an evaluative, but rather in a collaborative/therapeutic, role—when the relationship is less vertical and more horizontal—that patients will be more apt to reveal their most troubling thoughts, painful feelings, and dysfunctional interactions, for the purpose of working through their difficulties.

Because mental health professionals are in the truly privileged position of hearing the secrets of their therapy patients, many if not most of us have had the experience of sitting with someone contemplating parenthood, and, as therapists, we worry about the interpersonal environment—be it unstable, angry, narcissistic—into which the potential child would be brought. But this is all we can do—to hear our patients, to worry, and then to use this worry as a basis for confronting our patients with what they need to hear from us. Surely, no mental health professional is advocating for a world in which we prescreen men and women for psychological health prior to reproduction, and, surely, many of us would not be here today had our own parents been required to pass such a screening!

As a therapist, I sometimes feel like a peripheral character from the movie *Men in Black*. As a therapist, one has a dramatic interpersonal experience in a session (as the movie characters might have had to wrestle with an alien being), and then afterwards the Will Smith character (one of the eponymous men in black) takes out a small "zapper" and gives one's brain a painless zap that effectively clears the experience from awareness. Whatever a patient's psychological problems may be, whatever his or her relationship difficulties, if I happen to see this person outside the session, on the street or at a local school or place of worship, I will not reveal my private therapeutic experience with her. Similarly, if the patient happens to be a fertility patient, and if I see her sitting in the waiting room of the reproductive medicine clinic, the content of our private experience cannot show in my words, my expressions, or my gestures. Especially, the patient has to know that, if I happen to come across her reproductive endocrinologist, happen to end up sitting next to her RE in a meeting, her private therapeutic experience with me has been as good as zapped from my consciousness. A therapist must be capable, in other words, of keeping a secret and of compartmentalization. Ultimately, the function of evaluation notwithstanding, it is by being able to keep the secrets of others that we invite those others to open up to us for the purpose of working through the problems of their private lives.

WHEN THE DOUBTS ARE THE PATIENT'S

I have so far focused on situations where the therapist's perspective differs from that of the patient—at least on the surface—in that the therapist questions the readiness or motivation for parenthood of the patient, who seeks parenthood. But sometimes it is the patient who questions her own ability to parent.

Ellen K, age 30, suffered from premature ovarian failure; her husband demonstrated a severe male factor infertility. The couple did not want to use donor gametes and were in agreement to pursue domestic adoption to start a family. The Ks passed their home study and through an adoption lawyer had been able to connect with a birth mother who was due to deliver within months. Ms. K presented to me for psychotherapy upon learning that the birth mother was giving birth to a girl. Ms. K suddenly realized that, if she became the mother of a girl who was not extremely attractive, she could not tolerate it, possibly could not love the child. Ms. K had seen a picture of the birth mother and felt that she was reasonably, though not exceptionally, attractive. Ms. K herself was a very attractive woman, although she did not seem to dress or make herself up to accentuate her attractiveness.

I began questioning Ms. K about her relationship to her looks and the earliest origins of this relationship in her childhood. Did her mother, her father, tend to overvalue Ms. K's looks, at the expense of other, more internally based attributes? Ms. K described a history in which she, in fact, received some attention for being, first, an adorable child and then a lovely woman. The interaction with her parents, however, did not seem to be characterized by a predominant focus on her appearance. Ms. K's looks also meant that she received a fair amount of attention from men, but, notably, she was a fairly self-contained and quiet person and evidently not especially flirtatious. In any case, to whatever degree physical appearance was a focus for Ms. K, she herself pointed out that this issue had not overtly shaped her life. She felt that she had married her husband because he was a good and stable man who would be a good father and, though he was nice looking, she had not sought out the handsomest man she could find, nor necessarily the man most admiring of her looks. She worked as an accountant; she had not pursued a profession in which her appearance was paramount. In general, Ms. K was open to discussion of the origins of the presenting issue, although it was clear that this discussion did not inspire any major insights for Ms. K, nor did it alter one iota her feelings about the prospect of parenting a less than beautiful daughter.

I began to explore in more depth the adoption decision. Ms. K had known about her premature ovarian failure for several years and described a period of grieving the loss of her own genetic child and moving slowly toward adoption, a choice that became more solidified when it turned out that her husband had his own serious fertility problem. I asked Ms. K if she thought she might have the same hesitation or concern in regard to her child's appearance if she herself were giving birth to the child and were the child's genetic mother. The emphatic answer was no. Did she answer this way because she was certain that, if she were the genetic mother of the baby, this baby would be guaranteed to be beautiful? The emphatic answer here, too, was no. Ms. K spontaneously brought up instances of several people she knew who were themselves very attractive but who had children who were not especially good looking and she knew some unattractive people who had beautiful kids. Ms. K felt that, if it were she who gave birth to a daughter who was not very pretty, she could still, positively, accept the child.

For me, what seemed best to capture the nature of Ms. K's adoption anxiety was anxiety about "the other"—a form of xenophobia, if you will. We began to explore this aspect of Ms. K's psychology and its origins. Ms. K depicted her parents as fairly secretive people who liked to "keep to themselves." While Ms. K was growing up, the family seldom had company, neither extended family nor friends. Her parents encouraged her to play at home with her brothers, rather than invite friends over or go out to friends' homes. In recent years, both her mother and her father had been involved in ongoing disputes with their own family members (their siblings). Neither parent had especially approved of any of her boyfriends, and, when Ms. K originally became involved with her husband, both parents managed to find fault with him. Interestingly, regarding the adoption itself, Ms. K described her parents as positive and approving. She also mentioned that both were long aware of her inability to have a child and that both parents were "against" international adoption.

I interpreted Ms. K's fear that her soon-to-be-adopted child would be insufficiently attractive as an anxiety about the "not-me." A child genetically related to her, even if no great beauty, would still be in the "me" category, part of her. She feared what was not part of her. This may well be a normal anxiety that adoptive parents as well as parents through gamete donation need to confront and work through. In Ms. K's case, her level of trepidation threatened to derail the adoption.

Our therapeutic work in the area of Ms. K's psychological relation to the "other" seemed to do little to alter her feelings or her fears. In the transference/countertransference dynamic, I experienced her as being somewhat brittle, somewhat removed. She participated cooperatively in all our explorations and indicated an intellectual understanding of the connection between some of her family dynamics and her adoption anxieties. However, there was no "aha" experience for Ms. K, not even close. As her therapist, I would have felt gratified and relieved had she been able to make the connection between family experiences and current fears and then successfully let go of some of her worries. Instead, her attitude was that our discussions were mildly interesting to her and that she appreciated my wish to help her. But she nonetheless remained just as concerned that (a) her child would not be attractive enough and (b) this unattractiveness would prevent her from bonding appropriately with the child. No doubt Ms. K possessed hidden resistances to taking in my interventions. Suffice it to say that I found no way of effectively addressing these resistances, especially in the brief time allotted for us by circumstances (i.e., the impending birth).

As Ms. K approached the due date of her baby's birth mother, I maintained with her a neutral attitude, not because of some general stance I chose to take but because this was about all I could authentically muster with her. With other patients, whose anxieties about parenthood (whether through adoption or biologically) are clearly irrational and would not interfere with their forming a loving relationship with the child, I would not hesitate to label their irrational anxieties as such and take an actively reassuring role with them. With Ms. K, I simply could not take this stance. Countertransferentially, I was, in fact, worried that she would not be able to love the child in the way the child would need to be loved.

So, ultimately, I was worried, but not so worried that I felt moved to encourage Ms. K to walk away from the adoption. She herself did not choose to do this, and I suppose I did not feel enough alarm actively to question her choice. Whatever degree of guarded optimism I did experience about the impending adoption, I perhaps experienced because Ms. K did appear to be forthcoming with me. In part, I thought, because of a sense of disconnection and removal from me (which echoed the sense of disconnection from her prospective child), she seemed to feel no pressure at all to have me think highly of her or to see her in a certain way. Thus, I perceived that whatever she was telling me was the worst of what she felt. Granted, our therapeutic work seemed to do little to change what she felt, but I thought (and certainly hoped) that maybe at least part of the presenting situation was that Ms. K was more honest than the average person (honest with both herself and others) about some of her "ugly," unattractive feelings.

Approximately two months after Ms. K and her husband went off to another state to adopt their daughter, Ms. K brought her new baby in to meet me. Fortunately (for everyone concerned, and especially the child), it was clear to me that Ms. K was unreservedly in love with her daughter. Of course, I delicately brought up the issue of appearance, after all, the issue that had brought her in to see me. "Well, look how beautiful she is!" Ms. K exclaimed. Yes, her baby was adorable, but to my neutral eye, she was beautiful in the way that babies tend to be beautiful, not in some greater, superior way. As Ms. K saw it, she had lucked out. She had simply been fortunate enough to receive that beautiful baby she needed to have. She showed no sign of any insight into the origins of her presenting problem—her fear that she could not love the child. For me, on the other hand, Ms. K had ultimately proven herself to be capable of forming an attachment; from there, her appreciation of her child's beauty had flowed. It is no accident that we speak of faces "only a mother could love." Ms. K had become a mother, not just literally, but in the deeper sense. I was fortunate enough to be able to follow Ms. K every so often for a period of several years, and was relieved to see no sign of her presenting fears' becoming a reality.

The leap of faith that anyone must take in imagining that, by having a child, one will somehow be able to love the child in a "good-enough" way is a process that is intensified for those who must work really hard and wait really long to have a child. It is further intensified for those among us who require third parties in order to have this child. A therapist, as a witness to and sometimes facilitator of this process, may need to take a leap similar to that of the patient and trust that, for most who venture into parenthood, attachment will somehow happen. The research of Cowan and colleagues (Cowan and Cowan, 2002; Mikulincer et al., 2002) on attachment behavior and parenting shows us that there may be key psychological factors in parents-to-be that correlate with their children's subsequent emotional development. Fortunately, this research also points to early interventions in the couple's relationship that have improved the long-term outlook for families with potential problems in attachment.

Over the years, I have seen cases that were considered "at risk" for parenting, where attachment has nonetheless successfully occurred. I have seen a well-stabilized schizophrenic woman turn out to be a loving and reasonable mother to her child. I have seen a poor, uneducated couple with virtually no social support becoming unusually affectionate, patient, and concerned parents to their handicapped child. In contrast, I have also, however infrequently, observed situations where—in the absence of acute psychopathology, such as postpartum depression—parental attachment has been overtly lacking or inadequate. What has struck me especially about those cases is that the failure to attach emotionally was—or would have been—very difficult to predict, for I am talking about people, all middle class, seemingly "solid citizens," who otherwise presented in an ordinary, unremarkable, "normal" manner.

SUMMARY AND CONCLUSIONS

Motivation for parenthood always comprises a multiplicity of desires, some more wholesome than others. Persons procreating naturally are not subjected to evaluation of their motivations or their likely parenting abilities. In contrast, persons who seek assistance in conceiving a child are often referred for some kind of psychological consultation as part of their medical treatment, particularly if they require third-party reproduction (gamete donation or gestational carrier). Psychological consultation with reproductive patients is complicated by the emotional impact of infertility, as the stress of infertility tends to wreak havoc on psychological coping strategies. Whatever the manifold psychological factors that fuel the wish for a baby, mental health professionals should look carefully for the original, normal wish for a child that has set this whole process—the now arduous quest to procreate—in motion.

When patients are referred for psychological consultation as part of their reproductive treatment, the vast majority present themselves in a normative fashion, sending up no "red flags" that would indicate to the consultant that there is a serious problem in going forward with fertility treatment. On occasion, the psychological consultant does discover the presence of a serious problem that is apt to interfere with parenting—either a basic unwillingness to accept emotionally the planned reproductive treatment (such as the rejection of sperm donation by one partner) or the existence of serious psychopathology (such as substance abuse or domestic abuse). When such a problem surfaces, it becomes important to address this serious issue with the patients and to be prepared to recommend that patients delay conceiving a child until the problem is sufficiently ameliorated. Recommending delay entails empathizing with the patients' motivation to have a child while identifying the obstacles to adequate parenting and assisting the patients in overcoming these obstacles.

When it is neither the mental health professional nor the reproductive endocrinologist, but rather the patient, who questions his or her own prospective ability to parent, the mental health professional must be willing to immerse herself along with the patient in the patient's deepest anxieties about his or her inability to love, while maintaining a cautious optimism that the patient will likely be able to achieve this bond.

Psychologists and other mental health professionals tend to be good at understanding behavior that has already occurred, but a lot less good at predicting future behavior. That our predictive powers are limited underscores the importance of allowing people the freedom to pursue happiness by pursuing parenthood, as long as we as mental health professionals do not have compelling reasons to stand in their way.

REFERENCES

Cowan, P. A. & Cowan, C. P. (2002), Strengthening couples to improve children's well-being. *Poverty Res. News*, 3:18–20.

Mikulincer, D., Florian, V., Cowan, P. A. & Cowan, C. P. (2002), Attachment security in couple relationships: A systemic model and its implications for family dynamics. *Family Process*, 41:405–434.

3

WHEN THE THERAPIST
IS INFERTILE

Nancy Freeman

MY STORY

As luck would have it, I met and married my husband when I was 42 and discovered that I was pregnant twice during the first year of our relationship. After the second miscarriage, I was advised to pursue infertility treatment or adoption. Attempting to achieve pregnancy by using donor ovum was highly recommended by my physician, but, after such spontaneous pregnancies, I could not immediately give up the wish for a baby that would be a biological mix of my husband and me. However, after one failed in vitro fertilization treatment, we proceeded with preparations for ovum donation, and at this writing are waiting for an available donor.

MY EXPERIENCE OF INFERTILITY TREATMENT:
BACKGROUND TO CLINICAL MATERIAL

Between January and August of this year I went through a variety of treatments that required early morning examinations, blood tests, or both. For the first round of treatments in January, I rescheduled most of my patients in advance but had to do so at the last minute on at least one occasion. As I became familiar with the medical office routine, I was able to make all my morning appointments. Therefore, my infertility treatment did not interfere with patient schedules, a rare and lucky occurrence for me; when medical treatment requires missed appointments—or an altered manner of working (such as phone sessions or working from home), the sequelae are more profound and prolonged (Gerson, 1996). I am tempted to say there were minimal physical signs of what I was going through, but I know that what I was going through was enormously preoccupying.

As Rosen (this volume) suggests, the technology of infertility treatment (e.g., sonograms) complicates the patient's emotional reactions: she is asked to witness minute changes in her body displayed large on the sonogram screen and maintain a balanced, cautious view of the meaning of each microscopic development. This hyperawareness, which can extend to the woman's experience of her menstruation and more external changes in her body creates room for fantasies and magical thinking that link subtle physical sensations with the desire to make meaning, create hope, or counter superstitions. This sensitivity—physical, emotional, and cognitive—is both a distracting and an isolating experience. It is difficult to admit to oneself the range and intensity of fantasies and the intricate way in which they are linked with subtle or imagined physical experiences.

My memory of these months, during my hours with patients, is of a sense of relief from the relentless focus on myself. The days and weeks that preceded the miscarriages were most fraught with concern about my body. The in vitro fertilization cycle was a time filled with worry about my emotional state, in addition to an anxious awareness of changes in my body. At home, I felt intense, shifting moods, and I worried that my lability would distort my response to patients. I had the illusion that my office was a sanctuary from such emotional storms and believed that the effort of maintaining the status quo helped me feel most like myself during sessions. However, this self-control and dissociation held me apart from my experience, and consequently I felt less creative and spontaneous.

As Bromberg (1998) reminds us, dissociation can be seen as a defense against fragmentation of self-states. Dissociation protects, if only temporarily, the illusion of a coherent self. Like any contact with medical treatment, infertility attacks the core self (Stern, 1985), altering each patient's capacity for self-regulation (Beebe, Jaffe, and Lachmann, 1992). Self-regulation is a shorthand way of speaking of a person's multiple physical experiences of affective states, levels of arousal and activity, and the shifts between them (i.e., from sleep to alertness, from discontent to happiness). We perceive self-regulatory capacities when we notice a person's rhythms, moods, and gestures. In any contact between two people, each person's self-regulation combines with the interactive regulation of the dyad. Interactive regulation is another way of speaking of the organization of the dyad or system, that is, the mutual influence of each partner on the other (Beebe et al., 1992).

A much simplified example would be if self-regulation (i.e., one's capacity to feel calm or be able to listen attentively) is strained, there will be an impact on one's participation in the interactive regulation of the dyad (one could be less engaged or more intrusive), and a shift in the interactive regulation will similarly shift self-regulation. Shifts in self- and interactive regulation are particularly important in clinical work, as these combine with the range of nonverbal communication that occur in each dyad. Nonverbal communication is particularly relevant because it is the bedrock of knowing how to be with others, the "implicit relational knowing" or "coconstruction and taking in of another person" that evolves into internal object relations or psychic structure (Lyons-Ruth et al., 1998).

Clinicians are often aware of the effect on their own self-regulation and their own implicit relational knowing in the therapeutic process; this self-consciousness is even more present when the clinician is watchful of the effect of an obvious change in her self-regulation, such as comes with a life crisis.

How I responded to infertility treatment, specifically its impact on my sense of self, is connected to basic facts of my development, professional as well as personal. After I regained my usual sense of myself, I was aware that during this period of infertility I had become plagued by a sense of insecurity I felt I had outgrown earlier. My past internal dialogue had been dominated by feelings of inadequacy and questions about my behaviors. This dialogue created an awkward self-consciousness that was familiar and uncomfortable. During infertility treatment, this revivified internal experience influenced my self-regulatory capacities and, by extension, the balance of my attention to myself and others.

To summarize, it is useful to describe such changes in self-organization as variations in implicit relational knowing (Lyons-Ruth et al., 1998), as well as fluctuations in the capacity for intersubjectivity (Benjamin, 1988), or as a figure–ground movement between a sense of dependence and independence (W. Wilner, 2003, personal communication). Mitchell (2000) combined these ideas in his vision of four different modes of functioning, a structure of increasing organization that he used to compare different relational theories.

SOME MEANINGS OF INFERTILITY:

A ROADBLOCK TO ADULT DEVELOPMENT

Infertility treatment is complicated because it is about pregnancy and, by extension, about parenthood and the dynamic issues that lead people to create families with children or remain childless. Such issues may include idealization of one's family of origin or dreams of creating a more "perfect" family, both potential strategies to repair past trauma. The desire for children may derive from many different motivations, including a biological imperative, a responsibility to one's culture and ancestors, or a narcissistic wish. I found that infertility treatment highlighted every possible ambivalent feeling about having children, as each step in treatment requires a commitment—financial, physical, and psychological—to the goal of becoming a parent.

Each woman's response to infertility treatment is organized around her own cultural attitudes and beliefs about children, family, and adult development, as well as those of her partner and family. Infertility treatment forces each patient to confront ideas about her sense of self, identity, and future—through the lens of not having children or of having non-biological children. Infertility may be experienced as a prohibition: the patient has been told she can not proceed with the desire to be a parent, have a family, or generally accomplish adult developmental steps to reach maturity and generativity (Erikson, 1968). This sense of a life proscribed because of a physical limitation, often perceived as a defect, is possibly why researchers have found that the experience of infertility is as devastating as a diagnosis of AIDS or cancer (Domar, Zuttermeister, and Friedman, 1993).

In American culture, marriage and children, in different ways, also represent an end to adolescence and the emergence of a solidified adult sense of self. Reluctance to take these steps is the source of much sitcom humor in our culture. Married people and people with families are assumed to have separated more, or more adequately, from their families of origin. This societal norm also pervades clinical presentations, that stereotypically end with "fairy tale endings," accounts of how the patient got married or, even better, got married and had children (Chodorow, 2003, p. 2). Infertility flouts these cultural assumptions and propels the patient back onto the wrong side of the cliche: Is a woman without the capacity to bear a child doomed to childishness herself? Are her extended family disappointed and her immediate family inadequate? Is she deprived of an essential form of feminine power and prerogative?

Our society often seems to equate childlessness with negative characteristics, including selfishness, immaturity, or more essential values such as being cold, or withholding, or other variants of "not" maternal or "not" nurturing. Leibowitz (1996) eloquently articulates a range of such transference reactions from patients when they learn that she is a childless analyst. Because my entrance into the world of infertility followed my late marriage, I was already familiar with issues involved in being a childless, single analyst. Living as a childless married adult, like being a single adult, can require ongoing adjustments of ambivalent feelings, a dance between longings and satisfactions. The pleasures of companionship, romance, and professional life may shift in emphasis, from foreground to background, with complex negative emotional states, including shame, loneliness, and inadequacy, which distort one's sense of competency and coherence (Leibowitz, 1996).

Chodorow (2003) succinctly states that psychoanalysis has historically misunderstood the importance of pregnancy and motherhood in female development and also ignores the role of these events in adult development for both men and women. There appears more to be said about the mixed pressures of personal inhibitions, family dynamics, and assumptions about gender roles that contribute to the struggle of many intelligent, ambitious men and women to find life companions. Rosen (this volume) advocates the importance of confronting each denial: "If a patient has not mentioned childbearing fears/hopes/dreams and is in her thirties, I bring up the issue. I am not trying to steer the patient into bearing a child; instead, I am curious about the absence of thought and/or preparation about the topic." This analysis can lead to discussion of attachment issues, oedipal rivalries, and other common obstacles to parenting, as well as the identity issues, shame, and despair that can accompany a woman's struggle to change in the face of pressure from her biological clock.

Chodorow (2003) takes a particular stand on this dilemma, and her formulations are a welcome addition to a complex psychological problem (perhaps uniquely important to women in postfeminist worlds) that receives inadequate attention. Linking her current clinical observations with the theoretical framework she evolved in *The Reproduction of Mothering*, Chodorow (1978) asserts, "Motherhood begins internally in the conflictual, intense cauldron of childhood sexuality and object relations and is over determined, filled with fantasy, and complex: any woman's desire for children, whether immediately fulfilled, fulfilled belatedly, or never fulfilled, contains layers of affect and meaning" (p. 4). And further, "Motherhood is in conscious and unconscious fantasy first and foremost a gendered bodily, object-relational, and cultural experience for women" (p. 8).

Chodorow (2003) uses clinical examples to illustrate "an intrapsychic conflation of attacks on the maternal womb and [the patient's] womb and reproductive possibilities" (p. 4). She emphasizes the self-destruction hidden in the "nonreproduction of mothering," although she does not explicitly link the woman's conflictual relationship with her mother and older siblings to her unfulfilled dependency needs. This link is implied, however, in her clinical examples of mothers who were experienced as "too tired and weakened" by daughters later compelled to play out a "turning inward of deadening aggression against the reproductive body in the context of anger at the mother and siblings, and the denial of time passing" (p. 4). Chodorow does not fully explain why a sense of the mother's unavailability interferes with a woman's capacity to move on with her life. In other words, how does she get caught in the vacuum of timelessness?

I would suggest that the denial of time passing is linked with the care withheld by the mother or thought to have been provided to siblings. Timelessness evolves, in part, out of an experience of dependency: a person denies time as an adult because she is trying to hold the world still until she gets what she needed, wanted, or deserved as a child. This disavowed dependency translates for many single women (and men) into a false state of independence, a way of being on one's own that is essentially an effort to satisfy one's desire to be taken care of. It is also possible that timelessness is expressed as the hope for an infinite future, a time that seems to be always unfolding, its potential just beyond one's grasp. That hope is hard to give up.

An aspect of this disavowed dependency that further supports the sense of timelessness is the consequence that it is difficult to learn about the world when one is dependent (Wilner, 2003). It is possible that delayed motherhood occurs in the context of women's lives when they feel independent but are inhibited by dependency, a constriction that leads to a way of "not knowing things about the world." In this sense, a woman may remain particularly unaware of the impact of aging on fertility, despite many references to it in the media, or she may describe dating and negotiating relationships as mysterious activities for her, despite an active social and professional life. The unresolved dependency that interferes with a capacity to know things about the world may be reevoked in the regressive responses to the strain of infertility treatment. As feelings of dependency are revived, as they are in any medical treatment, the patient becomes less able to feel confident of what she knows about the world, and especially about herself as a woman. Rosen (this volume) identifies the "loss of one's prior notions of self" as the most significant loss in infertility. For myself, I felt, at times, that I had lost access to my secure, satisfied self and was instead stuck with a more anxious, critical self.

COUNTERTRANSFERENCE

The contemporary psychoanalytic view of transference, counter-transference, and therapeutic action generally conceives of the therapist as embedded in the therapy—for example, as one subjectivity in an intersubjective exchange (Benjamin, 1988), or a participant–observer (Levenson, 1991), a participant in a dyadic system of self- and mutual regulation (Aron, 1992; Beebe, Jaffe, and Lachmann, 1992), or a coconstructor of a cooperative frame of reference (Wolstein, 2000), to name only a few conceptualizations of the analytic relationship. Still, conversation about countertransference easily slips into debate over how the analyst uses his experience of himself and of the patient: does he speak of it, think about it, or unwittingly act on it? Variations of these options are explored in Gerson's (1996) eloquent collection of essays about the impact of life crises and life circumstances on therapists and their work. There is agreement that the myth of analytic anonymity has been dispelled and replaced with interest in the uses of countertransference as a therapeutic tool; however, differences remain in recommendations to the therapist in the midst of a life crisis.

If an analyst prefers to provide minimal information, mostly related to issues of the frame (i.e., details of how she will continue working), there is support for that position in the writings of Abend (1982), Dewald (1990), and Lasky (1990). This stance encourages the analyst to be wary of interfering with the patient's fantasy or exposing the patient to a kind of manipulation for the therapist's need.

Among analysts who have provided more information about their life circumstances, there is general consensus that doing so has increased the opportunities for analytic engagement. Leibowitz (1996) and Gerson (1996a) most emphatically state that it is the analysis of a patient's reactions to information about the analyst that becomes the field for the most rewarding analytic work. Gerson (1996b) posits that it remains difficult to explore the range of reactions to crises in the analyst's life, for a more fundamental reason than decisions about whether or not to speak about one's self. It is because analysts continue to experience a kind of "regret for our humanness, even as we are more open about our humanness" (p. xvii). Fortunately, there have always been analysts who could remind us that, however well intentioned, this is not a required posture.

In a review of theoretical descriptions of countertransference, Tauber (1954) wrote: "We cannot escape ourselves. This does not leave us condemned or judged, nor does it encourage relativism. What I regard as countertransference is when I feel and behave as I should or ought rather than as I am" (p. 64). An expansion of Tauber's emphasis on the therapist's capacity to use himself in therapy in the fullest and most natural direction can be found in Wolstein's (2000) conception of the impact of anxiety in the analyst. Wolstein's view is that anxiety makes the analyst act unwittingly like a caricature of his internal idealized analyst.

Wilner (1998) defines this perspective as focused on "what we might consider to be authentic and inauthentic analytic participation (p. 414). Wilner elaborates that when the analyst veers away from lived awareness, he can become mired in metaphors. Wilner suggests that an analyst may shift between experiential and metaphoric modes, an idea of shifting experience that is not unlike the shifting capacity for intersubjectivity, described by Benjamin (1988), that can lead to a collapse of relatedness and communication. Experiential relating, like intersubjectivity, is a fluctuating capacity, and, in this sense, countertransference interferes in waves of metaphoric relating that obscure aspects of experience. Both Wilner (1998) and Tauber (1954) link limitations in the analyst's capacity to experience, or, in Tauber's words "to achieve that degree of constructive spontaneity" (p. 64) to his potential reluctance to give and receive—to take things in.

I believe this is the sort of countertransference that is especially heightened when the therapist is in the throes of a life event. It is possible that the problem of infertility has a particular impact on the therapist's capacity to be open and authentic because infertility is shrouded in secrecy. In my case, when the medical treatment did not "visibly" disrupt the therapeutic setting, there were external motivations not to speak of it. Indeed, even as infertility treatment proceeds, the patient is confronted with additional taboos about sharing news of an early pregnancy.

The following clinical examples illustrate my shifting capacity to be open and authentic. I have borrowed terminology from Lyons-Ruth et al. (1998) and Stern et al. (1998) in an effort, like Beebe and Lachmann's (1994) and Mitchell's (2000), to apply an understanding of nonverbal communication, gained through infant research, to the adult therapeutic experience. I understand these concepts (implicit relational knowing, now moments, and moments of meeting) to be important elaborations of the concern for analytic authenticity and availability to experience championed by Tauber (1954), Wolstein (2000), and Wilner (1998). The first example, Ms. C, occurred chronologically earlier in the course of these past two years and represents a retreat from openness. My anxiety about my circumstances led me to retreat from experiential relating and created awkward, ultimately difficult interactions in my work with Ms. C that only gradually resolved in the course of the past year. In the case of Ms. E, my openness was more authentic and less disruptive.

CLINICAL WORK WITH MS. C

Over the two-year period, from my marriage to the present, I gained significant weight and was generally less active and more uncomfortable with my body than usual. I believe that some of my patients noticed my discomfort. It was intriguing that those who inquired directly about my state, asking specifically if I was pregnant, usually did so at a point when I was not pregnant, and most asked at a time when I was not actively involved in any kind of medical treatment. The exception occurred in my work with Ms. C.

C is a woman in her early 30s who has felt lonely and unable to form a significant romantic relationship for most of the five years that she has been my patient. She is the oldest of three children, and she played a significant part in raising her two younger brothers. Her parents, both schizoid, depressed people, divorced when she was about five years old, shortly after the birth of her youngest brother. At that time, her mother collapsed into a psychotic depression, and she has spent the rest of her life battling a serious paranoid delusional disorder. During C's childhood, her mother received no treatment, and the chaos in the home included her brothers' rageful and destructive behavior.

Remarkably, until their high school years, the children maintained an unspoken pact of secrecy that colluded with the denial of their mother's illness. Despite regular contact, her father never asked about the mother's emotional stability or the children's safety and well-being, nor did he, his second wife, or any other authority figure ever acknowledge the mother's condition or intervene to improve the quality of the family's life. C left her mother and brothers to live with her father during high school. She was productive in college and was helped by a psychologist to continue to separate from her mother, who was hospitalized for the first time while C was away from home. In the 10 years since her college graduation, C has maintained contact with her mother, tolerated her frequent psychotic communications, and kept track of her compliance with medications. She also is regularly in touch with her father and stepmother, despite their psychological remove and lack of warmth.

C has discovered her parents' weaknesses after years of colluding with their denial. Neither parent provided a real connection with her, one that would have allowed C to know them or feel known herself. Consequently, she is hypervigilant to how others reveal or hide themselves. C had had one other therapeutic experience before we met that ended in her rage at the therapist's withholding stance. We worked together for several years before the period I am reporting. We were frequently in a battle over her desire to know more about me and her insistence that she could not modulate her own mood or contain her anxiety without gestures of support and signs of closeness with me. C is intelligent, talented, and competent; in the years that I have known her, however, she has veered between adequate self-care and a capacity to work efficiently with others, and periods of schizoid withdrawal, somatic complaints, limited functioning, and a self-destructive use of sleep medication to dull her feelings of agitation and rage.

C and I live in the same neighborhood, and she knew that I was also single. In retrospect, I minimized the meaning of both my physical presence near her and the many fantasies she had about my life. These fantasies gave her the sense that she knew me or had discovered things about me on her own and out of my awareness. One evening during the spring, we saw each other on the street. I was walking with a man toward my apartment. In the weeks that followed, C was upset at the discovery that there was a man in my life and found it nearly impossible to grapple with her despair and envy. At the end of June, C and I were still in the throes of her rageful responses to me, when she noticed my wedding ring the day I returned to work after a very brief honeymoon.

C had an intense reaction to not having been told in advance about this change in my life or my move to a different apartment only slightly farther from her own. In the midst of her distress, she focused on her fear that a pregnancy would follow my marriage.

Her insistence that I tell her if I was pregnant unfortunately matched my inability, at that moment, to deny that I was pregnant. I had already experienced one miscarriage, and, as the second pregnancy maintained itself, I became caught up with my own superstitions. I experienced her questions as a demand for me to negate my experience, something I was unwilling to do, even partially, because of my own fears. I acknowledged that she had guessed correctly (that I was indeed pregnant), even though I understood she did not need to know about my pregnancy. Her subsequent fury was expectable given our recent struggles and the painful, disturbing facts of her history and personal dynamics. C could not tolerate this truth; in her fantasy she feared that a new family was in my future and would overshadow my concern for her. She also expected that marriage and children, and the love and care for her that they implied, would never be in her future. She had believed that my life offered her the possibility of a model for living alone. And now she felt betrayed, envious, and destructive.

C could not be soothed, and, although she wanted some kind of constant support from me (she left phone messages with urgent demands to help her feel better), the anguish she felt in my presence was intolerable. She experienced a serious decompensation and arranged for a brief hospitalization. However, she mobilized herself to find adequate outpatient treatment apart from contact with me. When I was contacted by other clinicians regarding her care, I learned that she was focusing on her rage at my marriage but seldom mentioned my pregnancy. We stayed in touch, usually on the phone, but occasionally in person over the next year. When we resumed our work, C could not speak much about her reaction to my pregnancy or her current thoughts about it, although I introduced the subject and tried to encourage her to talk.

Serendipitously, another chance encounter on the street led us to repair this breach. I passed her in our neighborhood while I was walking with friends and holding the hands of my friends' twin five-year-old daughters. I was able to ask her about the experience of seeing me on the street and to say again that I thought she might have been wondering what happened to my baby. C was unusually incoherent and hesitant to speak. She vaguely acknowledged that she thought "for a second" that the children were mine. Her capacity to blur reality—to ignore their size and age—I believe was an unconscious recognition that she knew I had not had a child. I told her that I had had a miscarriage and also suggested that I thought she might have known this (because she had seen me during the year). I added that I believed she had not spoken of it because she had been afraid that she had hurt me and destroyed my pregnancy. I stated simply that her anger had not caused my miscarriage.

C nodded; she was tearful, but mostly silent. This moment was pivotal and difficult to explain. It was, like the instance when I told C that I was pregnant, a "now moment." Stern and his colleagues (1998) emphasize that such a present, affectively charged moment "pulls the two participants fully into the present" (p. 304). Moreover, a now moment reorganizes the system, and then that change needs to be made sense of, with authentic responses from both analyst and patient, to become in Stern et al.'s language, "a moment of meeting" (p. 305). In this brief clinical vignette, it may be difficult to describe how different C's nodding, tearful response felt, and how unusual my commonplace explanation of my own experience sounded in the context of our recent history of intense confrontation. I suggest that both of these transitional moments included shifts in my countertransference amd my capacity to be authentic, which then supported shifts in C's way of being.

There is much more to this story for C, including her reaction to her siblings' births, events that precipitated dramatic events in her family, and her disappointments in her parents', her therapists', and my own inability to mother her. However, there was a directness and an intimacy to our connection, and I felt her relax in a profound way.

CLINICAL WORK WITH MS. E

E is a single woman in her 50s whose life has been organized around the sequelae of a congenital endocrine condition that was untreated in childhood. In adulthood, her condition was complicated by related gynecological problems, including polycystic ovaries and fibroid tumors. To alleviate her intense symptoms, she had a hysterectomy at age 47 during the third year of our six years of working together. Unfortunately, she continues to struggle to regulate her response to synthetic estrogen, with periodic flare-ups of menopausal symptoms.

E's endocrine condition caused her to enter puberty at age eight years, and her family was notably insensitive to her experience. Owing to her condition, she appeared years older than her chronological age because she developed breasts, hips, and increased stature. She feels that there was always "a gap" between her internal age and others' perceptions of her. As a girl maturing before her peers, she felt she was "too sexual," and she labeled those feelings as wrong and unnatural. She had already begun to shut down, to avoid her sexuality, when her peers started to develop. She describes herself as "never having caught up," and sees this as the source of her trouble establishing an adult sexual life.

E's father, an artist, died nearly 10 years earlier, after suffering since E's teens from a congenital, deteriorating condition of his esophagus. Her mother is an energetic octogenarian who still works. E most often describes her mother as tending to minimize anything negative, especially her husband's illness and E's physical condition. In the years following E's father's death, her gynecological symptoms increased, which seemed in part related to her identification with him, but was plausibly the result of hormonal changes connected to her age and medical condition. Despite obvious intelligence and competence at work, she continues to see herself as adolescent, unable to take care of the details in her life, and, owing to her inexperience, unlikely to find love. Her sense of herself as damaged is seemingly intractable, despite our years of work and the many years of analytic work and weekly psychotherapy she has had with other clinicians.

When she began treatment with me, her life was consumed with medical appointments, and she filled sessions with complaints as well as specific medical questions that I could not answer. Although it was obvious that she was suffering many physical symptoms, she seemed predominantly psychologically fragile and unable to function. She was panicked almost monthly by the fear of heavy bleeding and what she perceived to be the continual threat of hemorrhage or an emergency hysterectomy. She called her doctors and her mother frequently with hysterical demands that they act immediately to help her. Her life was a struggle to have her physical complaints taken seriously. Her doctors seemed so frustrated by the persistence of her complaints that it appeared to me that her medical care might be compromised.

Following her complicated adjustment to the hysterectomy, E. was referred to a specialist who confirmed that she was often very accurate in her sense of even slight shifts in estrogen levels. This validation of her experience was very important to her and to our discussion of her symptoms. Her situation calls up many questions about the interaction of mind and body. We have discussed how lapses in her capacity for intersubjectivity, especially fluctuations of her denigrating attitude toward herself, were mirrored in the objectification of her body. When she feels herself to be inadequate, she describes herself as a cluster of symptoms; when she presents herself as impossible to soothe or inaccessible to hope for the future, she identifies herself as defective and incurable. The years since her hysterectomy have involved gradual shifts in her capacity to accept and accommodate her chronic medical condition. She has dramatically changed her behavior with medical doctors, especially the frequency of her appointments. She has also made real changes in her work life and taken on more responsibility despite intense anxiety about her ability to work when her she has physical discomfort. She has begun to compete with colleagues, to be assertive, and to feel comfortable with her increased authority.

E vacillates between a seemingly naïve, confused adolescent presentation (in this mode she sees me as a maternal figure) and a more mature persona, confident in her own style of dress and with cultured tastes and interests, who relates to me as a peer. Over the past six months, E intermittently raised the subject of ending treatment. She has expressed frustration that her sense of herself as flawed has not shifted. She has trouble regulating her self in response to interactions with supervisors and difficult colleagues. Both anger at perceived slights by others and fear of being found wrong or unprepared often override her capacity to make sense of the corporate system in which she works.

In the course of talking about termination, E had a flare up of physical symptoms reminiscent of her discomfort years ago. Her hormone levels were off; her estrogen was very low despite the high amounts of synthetic estrogen she was taking. She tried again to explain to me the overpowering feeling of being out of control, the waves of emotional lability and depression that felt intolerable to her. The intersection between her physical complaints and her psychological reality continued to confound me; I had a new perspective on her experience, however, after I had completed the in vitro fertilization treatment. In the course of taking extra hormones, I felt intense mood swings and had the clear sense, as E has described over the years, that the lability was controlled by hormone levels and had nothing to do with my psychological reality.

After she described her increased symptoms, E was surprised that I told her I really did think I understood her, and I explained that I too had had similar experiences in the past year while pursuing infertility treatment. E presented a somewhat frightened and deferential initial response. She asked only what I was taking and believed I had said that I was currently undergoing treatment. Then she rallied her more competent self and pronounced that she had believed all along that I did not fully credit her physical experience. She had known that I ultimately believed her complaints were intricately connected to "psychological issues." We spoke further of the differences between empathy and actually sharing experiences, a discussion that seemed to touch, but glide over, her frequent complaint that no one could cure her or understand why she found it so difficult to go on without being made whole or unafflicted. It was also interesting that after I admitted to having infertility treatments, E asked me about my marriage for the first time; she admitted that she had not noticed that I was wearing a wedding band. I had not noticed the degree to which she wanted to have us both stay the same, the way we were when we met.

There was an authenticity in this exchange that we rarely experienced together, in the midst of her usual complaints and my frequent confusion about how to help her. She had accepted the reality that she thought I did not understand her physical complaints, much as she had accepted her parents' disregard for her medical condition since childhood. E waited, as if time were not passing, for me to change my mind. E, and I have just begun to discuss what it meant for her to wait for me to catch up to her reality or what difference she feels now that I have shared some of her experience and understand her physical complaints better. The "now moment" that occurred with E became a "moment of meeting" as we linked her readiness to end treatment with her growing confidence in understanding herself, regardless of how she is misunderstood by others, including me. E continues to struggle with her own experience of timelessness, although I may see her in a new light, where she occasionally joins me but mostly she is looking forward to the time when she will consistently see herself as changed.

CONCLUSION

I pursued infertility treatment in my early 40s, following two miscarriages that occurred shortly after I was married for the first time. My marriage helped me experience (or coincided with a period in which I could experience) being myself with less self-consciousness than I had ever felt before (or at least not since some halcyon days of my youth). I gave up the harsh self-criticism, the periodic intense experience of shame that characterized my struggle to mature. In short, I accepted myself as I was and was joyful in my new-found comfort with myself. Infertility treatment challenged these hard-won self-states. The challenge to create a baby and the repeated experiences of loss and disappointment uniquely threatened my sense of competence, confidence, and self esteem.

I was frequently preoccupied with what I did and what I said. I also felt less aware of my experience in sessions with patients, a retreat that left me feeling uncreative and less playful. In my anxiety, I was too quick to answer a patient's question about myself and was unable to contain her experience of learning about my life. I was most aware of this difference as it shifted and I was again capable of being authentic, engaged, and containing of my patient's rage and my own feelings of inadequacy.

As I have felt able to be more in contact with my own experience, I have become more interested in analyzing myself and my patient's feelings about mothers, babies, and time. Leibowitz (1996) describes her increased curiosity about what it would be like to have children and how her interactions with patients would be different. I have found myself responding to neo-Kleinian theory (Mitrani, 2001), engaged by the investigation of mothers, indeed, even by the use of the verb "to mother." I wonder what my patients may think of what feels to me like a new way of inquiring about how they may need mothering. I am not, I believe, substituting or sublimating my wish to be a mother of a real baby, but I may have begun to experience myself as a mother in this way, a way I may have found in the course of learning about infertility.

REFERENCES

Abend, S. (1982), Serious illness in the analyst: Countertransference considerations. *J. Amer. Psychoanal. Assn.*, 30:365–375.

Aron, L. (1992), Interpretation as expression of the analyst's subjectivity. *Psychoanal. Dial.*, 2:475–507.

Beebe, B., Jaffe, J. & Lachmann, F. (1992), A dyadic systems view of communication. In: *Relational Perspectives in Psychoanalysis*, ed. N. Skolnick & S. Warshaw. Hillsdale, NJ: The Analytic Press.

——— & Lachmann, F. (1994), Representation and internalization in infancy: Three principles of salience. *Psychoanal Psychol.*, 11:127–165.

Benjamin, J. (1988), *The Bonds of Love*. New York: Pantheon Books.

Bromberg, P. M. (1998), *Standing in the Spaces: Essays on Clinical Process, Trauma, and Dissociation*. Hillsdale, NJ: The Analytic Press.

Chodorow, N. J. (1978), *The Reproduction of Mothering*, 2nd ed. Berkeley: University of California Press.

——— (2003), "Too late": Ambivalence about motherhood, choice and time. *J. Amer. Psychoanal. Assn.*, 51:1181–1198.

Dewald, P. (1990), Serious illness in the analyst: Transference, countertransference and reality responses—and further reflection. In: *Illness in the Analyst*, ed. H. J. Schwartz & A. L. Silver. Madison, CT: International Universities Press, pp. 75–98.

Domar, A., Zuttermeister, P. & Friedman, R. (1993), The psychological impact of infertility: A comparison with patients with other medical conditions. *J. Psychosom. Obstet. & Gyn.*, 14:45–52.

Erikson, E. (1968), *Identity, Youth, and Crisis*. New York: Norton.

Gerson, B. (1996a), An analyst's pregnancy loss and its effect on treatment: Disruption and growth. In: *The Therapist as a Person: Life Crises, Life Choices, Life Experiences, and Their Effects on Treatment*, ed. B. Gerson. Hillsdale, NJ: The Analytic Press, pp. 55–70.

———— (1996b). *The Therapist as a Person: Life Crises, Life Choices, Life Experiences, and Their Effects on Treatment*, ed. B. Gerson. Hillsdale, NJ: The Analytic Press, pp. xi–xii.

Lasky, R. (1990), Keeping the analysis intact when the analyst has suffered a catastrophic illness: Clinical considerations. In: *Illness in the Analyst*, ed. H. J. Schwartz & A. L. Silver. Madison, CT: International Universities Press, pp. 177–197.

Leibowitz, L. (1996), Reflections of a childless analyst. In: *The Therapist as a Person: Life Crises, Life Choices, Life Experiences, and Their Effects on Treatment*, ed. B. Gerson. Hillsdale, NJ: The Analytic Press, pp. 71–88.

Levenson, E. (1991), *The Purloined Self*. New York: Contemporary Psychoanalysis Books.

Lyons-Ruth, K. & Members of the Change Process Study Group (1998), Implicit relational knowing: Its role in development and psychoanalytic treatment. *Infant Mental Health J.*, 19:282–289.

Mitchell, S. A. (2000), *Relationality: From Attachment to Intersubjectivity*. Hillsdale, NJ: The Analytic Press.

Mitrani, J. L. (2001), *Ordinary People and Extra-Ordinary Protections*. East Sussex: Brunner-Routledge.

Stern, D. N. (1985), *The Interpersonal World of the Infant*. New York: Basic Books.

———— & Members of the Change Process Study Group (1998), The process of therapeutic change involving implicit knowledge: Some implications of developmental observations for adult psychotherapy. *Infant Mental Health J.*, 19: 300–308.

Tauber, E. S. (1979), Countertransference reexamined. In: *Countertransference*, ed. L. Epstein & A. Feiner. New York: Aronson, pp. 59–69.

Wilner, W. (1998), Experience, metaphor, and the crucial nature of the analyst's expressive participation. *Contemp. Psychoanal.*, 34:413–443.

Wolstein, B. (2000), Interview with Irwin Hirsch and Benjamin Wolstein. *Contemp. Psychoanal.*, 36:187–232.

4

THE THERAPIST'S NEGATIVE PRECONCEPTIONS ABOUT INFERTILITY TREATMENT

Linda D. Applegarth

$\mathcal{M}$edical knowledge and technology have advanced at a seemingly breakneck speed. Specifically, there have been significant changes in the expectations, hopes, and opinions of patients as well as the medical and scientific community about what the assisted reproductive technologies (ARTs) can and should offer. In the 20 years that I have specialized in the psychology of reproductive health care and infertility, I have seen the minds of patients and professionals change just as rapidly as the growth of the medical technology itself.

For example, in the early years of in vitro fertilization (IVF) the technology allowed women, usually age 35 or younger, with blocked or missing Fallopian tubes, the opportunity to achieve pregnancy using their eggs and their husbands' sperm. In some cases, men with ogliospermia (low sperm count) could also take advantage of IVF since the eggs were inseminated in a petri dish, eliminating the need for many sperm to compete for a single egg. It all seemed so simple and straightforward then; in vitro fertilization was a medical technology to help a young, married, heterosexual couple have a baby together.

Although the Roman Catholic Church and conservative "right to life" organizations were expressly opposed to the development of this technology either on the grounds that it did not include the "conjugal act' or was considered to be tampering with nature and God's will, most people seemed generally neutral or positive about this new way of assisting infertile couples. Twenty-five years later, millions of babies have been born through in vitro fertilization and its related technologies, and the treatment is now seen as a standard of care for infertility.

Although reproductive technologies have been significantly improved and refined over the past two and a half decades, they still continue to be highly stressful as well as emotionally and financially disruptive medical treatments for most people. Because this sophisticated medical technology offers no guarantee of success, the psychosocial data frequently allude to depression and anxiety along with feelings of guilt, social isolation, anger, and helplessness for couples undertaking these procedures.

NEW CHALLENGES TO THE PSYCHOTHERAPIST

Initially, the role of the mental health professional was to provide emotional support and guidance to infertile persons as they struggled to build their families. Some patients asked for education, understanding, and symptom relief; others wished to explore more fully intrapsychic issues and injuries along with the psychodynamics of relationships with partners and family members. Indeed, from the psychotherapist's point of view, it all seemed straightforward then and appropriate to our training and expertise. We were—and often still are—asked to help assuage the pain and fear and uncertainty that go along with being infertile.

As the assisted reproductive technologies have expanded and changed, however, so have our roles. Specific technologic developments have made this so: embryo freezing (cryopreservation), the ability to diagnose genetic problems in embryos (preimplantation genetic diagnosis [PGD]), the ability to inject mechanically a single sperm into a human egg (intracytoplasmic sperm injection [ICSI]), ovum donation, embryo donation, and the ability of a woman to carry another couple's offspring (gestational surrogacy) have generally created greater opportunities for couples to have healthy children. No longer can we insulate ourselves from 21st-century reproductive medicine and sit behind closed doors with our grieving childless patients who long for a biological baby but know that they must also consider adoption as the alternative parenting option. Ironically, assisting our patients in coming to terms with the real losses of infertility has become increasingly difficult. The advent of assisted reproductive technology has meant that the losses themselves have also become more and more illusive. Just as one treatment door closes, another opens. Patients can often dodge the painful narcissistic injuries that are intrinsic to the inability to have a biological child.

Today we, as psychotherapists and mental health professionals, are asked to go "where no therapist has gone before." We must consider a wide range of medical treatments and options—actively sought out by patients and encouraged and supported by physicians, embryologists, and clinics—that can allow our patients to avoid confronting and mourning the many real losses normally associated with the inability to have a child. Some of these medical possibilities frankly offer excellent family-building opportunities for people; others, however, create grave and difficult moral and ethical conflicts for a psychotherapist. These ethical dilemmas can cause the therapist to have negative feelings about the technology but, even worse, about the patient(s) involved. These conflicts often go well beyond political or religious conservatism or liberalism and strike at the heart of what appears to be an "anything goes as long as I get what I want" mentality on the part of the patient and the medical community.

As psychologists and psychotherapists, I and many of my colleagues are confronted on a regular basis with requests to meet with individuals and couples who, with apparently little or no financial restraints, wish to have a child by using medical technology in what we consider to be a self-serving or ethically questionable way. Infertility centers and patients alike may not use our services as a way of better understanding the complex psychosocial issues involved for decision-making or for evaluating the psychological and emotional appropriateness of the parties involved (recipients, gamete donors, surrogates, and families). Rather, we may be called on to "rubber stamp" an arrangement so that something can be put in writing, for liability reasons, affirming that a mental health professional was consulted. This situation may reflect the fact that infertility treatments in this country are often considered an "industry" where the goal is financial success just as much, if not more than, solid, successful pregnancy rates. The difficulty arises for mental health professionals when we suddenly find ourselves being compensated for providing a psychosocial clean bill of health rather than for our honest clinical judgment, input, and expertise.

Some years ago, my colleagues and I worried, ironically, that we would be turned into the "gatekeepers" whose role would be to determine who was eligible to receive treatment and who was not. While this occasionally continues to be the case, often it is not. All too often, in the highly competitive United States arena of reproductive medicine, mental health professionals are consulted to lend further credibility and justification to a procedure rather than to question the applicability or appropriateness of that procedure for specific patients.

This dilemma, which has both ethical and clinical components, often leads to feelings of discomfort, resentment, or distress on the part of the therapist. To work effectively in this environment, it is critical that these conscious and unconscious feelings be acknowledged and addressed. Often how a therapist feels about the patient(s) is a barometer of how other people also feel about the patient. Although this type of countertransference provides germane clinical data about how the patient relates to the outside world, negative affect on the part of the therapist may also be, in part, a projection of feelings that the therapist has toward the referring physician or infertility clinic. These feelings may include resentment or indignation.

In an effort to clarify further some of the negative preconceptions and biases that psychotherapists practicing in the field of infertility must confront and deal with, I offer a number of case studies. These vignettes cover a number of difficult and often controversial areas that call upon us to consider our personal values and clinical skills.

ANECDOTAL CASE STUDIES ELICITING NEGATIVE THERAPIST RESPONSES

Sylvia

Sylvia presented as an attractive, outgoing 34-year-old Caucasian female. She reported that she was approximately 14 weeks pregnant and had been referred to me by her obstetrician because of depression and ambivalence about the pregnancy. At our first meeting, she reported that she was very happily married to a successful banker. Both had agreed to have only one child. She had told no one, except her husband and her father, that she was pregnant. Apparently, Sylvia had had no trouble conceiving. Her reasons for not telling others of her pregnancy were, she said, that she hated being pregnant and was not sure she wanted a child. Sylvia added that she had felt especially pressured by women friends to have children.

She described herself as a child of divorce. She had an older sister who had a long history of clinical depression and substance abuse. Sylvia was highly ambivalent about women. When she was still a toddler, her mother left the family, and her father raised her. Sylvia had been very close to her stepmother, who died several years previously. She was estranged from her mother and often referred to her only as "my biological mother." Managing her sister's mental health problems had been extremely difficult for her father and for her. Sylvia stated that part of her depression came from the concern that her fetus was female.

She staunchly believed that mental illness was a genetic trait carried by the females in her family, and she indicated that she planned to have amniocentesis to learn not only about the health of the fetus, but also about the gender. Approximately one month later, following the results of the amniocentesis, Sylvia learned that she was pregnant with a healthy female. Several days later, after Sylvia located a physician who was willing to perform a later-term abortion, the pregnancy was terminated. Although her husband apparently supported her decision, only her father, a radiologist, accompanied her for the abortion. She stated that she did not want to make the termination "too real" for her husband.

Sylvia and I met regularly following the abortion to explore her feelings about it as well as about motherhood in general. She began working part time, and her depression lessened substantially. Ultimately, she decided to seek out a fertility clinic that would do PGD for gender selection for a "nonmedical reason." After doing PGD on several IVF cycles as well as natural and medicated IUI cycles (using "microsort"—a procedure designed to select out sperm of only one gender), Sylvia failed to conceive after a year of treatment. Although she was distressed when the treatment cycles failed, she tended to bounce back quickly, citing her work and psychotherapy as reasons. She also noted that she was aware that she was capable of having a full life with or without a child. Several physicians she consulted agreed that she was in premature ovarian failure. Ovum donation was recommended. Surprisingly, Sylvia adjusted easily to the idea—in part, because she felt that "my gene pool is not that great, anyway." However, she insisted that, in order to move ahead with third-party reproduction, she must also have gender selection with PGD to have a male child—despite using donated eggs.

Sylvia presented several issues to me that led to negative feelings on my part. As her psychotherapist, I felt that the abandonment by her mother was a key to understanding not only Sylvia's ambivalence about motherhood, but also her unrelenting demand to have a male child. Her intense ambivalence and her willingness to kill a healthy fetus left me initially with concern about her ability to be a parent.

After two years of therapy, Sylvia was unwilling to explore in depth her feelings about this issue, although she easily admitted that her poor relationship with her mother was at least one reason she preferred to have a boy. More salient for me was working with someone who chose to abort a healthy fetus simply because it was not the desired gender and then to use the ARTs to determine the preferred gender of the child. Most distressing was the need to use preimplantation diagnosis on embryos that did not contain her genetic material and would thus have little chance of inheriting the mental illness that Sylvia dreaded. At this stage, the preimplantation genetic diagnosis would be used purely for the purpose of sex selection. The decision to do this seemed an effort to control her environment—past, present, and future. It appeared to be an effort unconsciously to prevent the possibility that she, as a mother, might also reject or abandon a daughter. In addition, it appeared that her expectations about parenting a male child might be quite unrealistic, particularly because there were no guarantees that the child could ever meet those expectations.

Although progress with Sylvia was slow, I experienced with interest how much I enjoyed my work with her. She was often open about her feelings and had a very endearing way of interacting with me. This style was apparently defensive, but her charm and sense of humor often kept me connected to her. When she introduced material that would otherwise create feelings of aversion or rejection on my part, I found myself feeling neutral or even sympathetic to her cause.

Her increased comfort with the idea of parenthood was also noteworthy, as she became clear about what was truly important in life to her and her husband. Ironically, Sylvia would often talk about her 16-year-old niece (the daughter of her divorced older sister) for whom she felt great love and affection. She demonstrated the ability to be parental and was able to set clear boundaries with the teenager. Sylvia had also had a very warm and positive relationship with her stepmother—a woman who had been instrumental in raising her. These factors ultimately played an important role in Sylvia's understanding of the role of parenthood in her life but did not dissuade her from her determination to have a male offspring. The progress she made in treatment and the efforts she made to become clear about her priorities helped me contain many of my own negative, rejecting feelings about her and the way in which she was using assisted reproductive technology for her own purposes.

Several months later, Sylvia was matched to an egg donor. Two healthy "male" embryos were transferred, but Sylvia did not become pregnant. Although Sylvia has continued in treatment with me, it is likely that she and her husband will no longer seek to become parents. She seems resolved on this issue and has stated on several occasions that she feels she and her husband did all they could. She continues to focus on family and career issues.

Mary and Jeff

Jeff presented to the scheduled appointment on time; Mary, however, was 20 minutes late. She said that she had been tied up in a meeting at work and was unable to get to the appointment. Both were well dressed and controlled and appeared confident. Although they were polite, Mary expressed some displeasure about having to meet with me because "there's really no point." They had agreed to meet with me only because their doctor, a reproductive endocrinologist in private practice, had requested the meeting.

The primary purpose in the meeting was to discuss the couple's desire to do in vitro fertilization and freeze the resulting embryos for future use. Jeff, age 37, stated that he was eager to have children. Mary, age 35, was heavily involved in her career in marketing. She indicated that she did not want children for at least five years, if at all. She added, however, that she was aware that her fertility would begin to decline over the next several years. After some discussion between them, Mary and Jeff contacted a fertility specialist. They asked to have in vitro fertilization performed within the next several months; and, at some time when it was more convenient, they would attempt to achieve a pregnancy using the stored cryopreserved embryos. Both Mary and Jeff believed that their request was both practical and efficient.

The issue that led to my negative feelings toward this couple was their sense of entitlement. This sense stemmed not only from their belief that they would have children only when it was completely convenient but also that the medical technology should be fully available to them. There was no indication that Mary and Jeff were infertile; they believed that they should have access to assisted reproductive technologies as a convenience. I was struck not only by their arrogance, but also by the couple's lack of affect. They seemed formal and businesslike in their interactions with me but also with one another. Because their physician was reluctant to work with them, I suggested that we meet together for four additional sessions. This recommendation followed some history-taking that allowed me to gain some insight into the marriage and to learn more about their families of origin.

By the end of the third session, it became clear that there were significant marital conflicts and issues that had never been articulated or addressed by either partner. Nonetheless, my initial emotional response to this couple was that of moral outrage. There was a sense that they were too busy and too important to be bothered with parenthood. The available medical technology thus fed their narcissism and arrogance.

By the end of the fifth session, the couple also recognized that cryopreserving their embryos was avoiding dealing with divergent life goals and aspirations that included, but was not limited to, children and parenting. In essence, the couple was attempting to keep their relationship "frozen" rather than "alive and growing." Their efforts to control completely their environments and their futures left them distant and isolated from one another. The couple's therapy has continued with a focus on striking a comfortable balance among careers, marriage, and parenthood. Mary and Jeff's willingness to explore feelings and issues has significantly mitigated my own negative countertransference.

Although this case resolved itself positively for the patients and for me, it is likely that an increasing number of educated and ambitious couples may wish to freeze embryos. They would thus be able to postpone parenthood so that "advancing maternal age" ceases to be a concern. Parenthood could ultimately become a matter of convenience for busy couples who might have difficulty fitting children into the current context of their lives. Troubling to a therapist may be not only the sense of entitlement that goes along with this desire, but also the ethical concern that these couples would be creating human embryos that might never be used. Furthermore, we all may ask whether assisted reproductive technology should be used for this purpose. Certainly, the original intent behind its development was to offer a treatment alternative for infertile couples who might not otherwise be able to conceive their own children. What is viewed as the misuse or abuse of this medical technology may create an array of negative feelings for the therapist toward potential patients as well as the providers of the technology.

Rebecca

Rebecca was a 40-year-old, single Latina. At the time she was referred, she was working as a file clerk in a large company. Although her salary was low, the company provided excellent benefits and would cover three IVF treatments. Often, before proceeding with assisted reproductive technology, single women are referred for a psychosocial consultation and possible counseling, if necessary. Unique to this case was that Rebecca, having been born with mild cerebral palsy (CP), was partially bound to a wheelchair. Although she was able to work and live independently, she lived near her parents and 32-year-old sister (engaged to marry), who provided ongoing emotional and physical support. They would often assist her with food preparation and personal hygiene. Aside from her CP, Rebecca was reported to be in good health.

Rebecca wanted to become a single mother but, because of her advanced age, would have to do IVF to optimize her chances of pregnancy. She stated emphatically that she was uncomfortable using an anonymous sperm donor. Instead, she had the idea of using the sperm of a 52-year-old married workmate, with whom she had briefly discussed this possibility. Although he agreed, he said that he would not inform his wife of this decision since it was "none of her business."

The reproductive endocrinologist that Rebecca consulted expressed uncertainty about her request and referred her to a psychologist. Although the physician was willing to move ahead as long as the sperm was quarantined for the required six-month time period, she also reported some concern about Rebecca's financial and physical limitations. The physician's referral to me included the statement, "I'm willing to go ahead with this if you say it's OK."

Rebecca was late for the appointment because she had to be driven by an aunt, who had taken off work to help Rebecca get to the meeting. Notwithstanding her physical disability, Rebecca was intelligent and articulate. She stated that she had always hoped to marry and have children. She now realized that marriage was unlikely, but she desperately wanted a child in her life. She was unclear as to how she would support herself and a child but said that she knew her parents, sister, and other relatives would help with child care. She noted, "They all just want me to be happy." Rebecca also said that the idea of using an anonymous sperm donor was "repulsive" to her because she would probably get an unattractive, offensive donor.

On the other hand, she said that she would not expect the known sperm donor (workmate) to have anything to do with the potential child. She was ready to move forward as soon as possible because she knew that "everything will work out fine." Rebecca added that she was dismayed to learn that the donor's sperm would have to be tested and quarantined for the six-month period.

As the mental health professional involved in this referral, I felt immediate discomfort. Even before meeting with Rebecca, I felt the need to sort out my negative feelings about Rebecca's request as well as my anger toward the referring physician. Clearly, I was being put in an extremely difficult position by indirectly being asked to make this situation work to all parties' satisfaction. I was also being asked to collude with these parties in supporting the potential sperm donor's infidelity and betrayal of his wife.

When I met with Rebecca, it became clear that, despite her intelligence and motivation to parent, she was extremely naïve about what would be involved in the medical process as well as what it might mean to raise a child alone. Her financial resources were very limited, and I was asked to reduce my fee to meet with her. The entire situation overwhelmed me and led me to feel resentment toward all the parties involved.

Ultimately I agreed to meet with Rebecca for four evaluative sessions. My goal was to educate her about what would be required of her as a parent and to inform her of some of the potential legal ramifications of using a known sperm donor. I also told her, as well as her physician, that I would not participate in any donor situation that did not include the consent of the donor's wife. I felt that, until these issues were addressed and clarified, it was impossible to help Rebecca deal with her feelings of loss and disappointment regarding her dream of being a wife and mother. This clarification also allowed me to deal with my own feelings of anger and resentment for I could begin to feel less responsible for "fixing" the situation for everyone. Acknowledging my own values and ethical limitations could only beneficially serve the patient.

During the third session with Rebecca, she gave permission to have her family members (parents and sister) invited to meet with us. It seemed critical to gain an understanding of how supportive her family would be if she were, indeed, to have a child. Her family was, in fact, very open to the idea. However, they insisted that, if she were to become pregnant, she would have to move back home with them so that Rebecca could be better supported physically, financially, and emotionally. They were openly and strongly opposed to the idea of her using her friend at work as a donor. Although Rebecca was resistant, she agreed that the circumstances with this man could potentially be complicated. She was willing to get more information and explore her feelings about using an anonymous donor. Rebecca and I met for an additional two sessions to discuss anonymous sperm donation. Her lifelong physical disability and control issues appeared to play a role in her negative fantasies about an anonymous donor. Our brief work together also involved a discussion of how she might share information about conception with the potential offspring.

Although my involvement in this case was less than complete, I was able to deal with my negative preconceptions by clarifying my own ethical and treatment limitations. These limitations needed to be expressed to both my patient and to the treating physician. It also seemed imperative, in this particular case, to understand and access the family support system before making valid recommendations about proceeding with treatment.

Carol and Sam and Molly

After two years of infertility treatment, Carol and Sam were told that they would need to move to ovum donation or adoption if they were to become parents. The couple, both in their early 40s, had been married for three years. Carol had been married briefly in her early 20s but this was Sam's first marriage. Both were successful attorneys, very eager to become parents. They reported that they were very happily married and wished to share their love and happiness with a child.

The couple reluctantly decided that ovum donation was the most comfortable parenting option for them. They were firm, however, that they were unwilling to use an anonymous donor. After several months of consideration, Sam and Carol approached their physician with a request to use Carol's 21-year-old niece, Molly, as a donor. Carol stated that she very much wanted her gene pool "in the mix" and felt that Molly, her older sister's daughter, was both intelligent and a good physical match.

Molly had recently graduated from college and had expressed her desire to attend graduate school in history. Her mother had spoken to her about Carol and Sam's infertility and need for donated eggs. Molly did not really know what was involved but expressed a willingness to help "Aunt Carol." Molly was then told that, in return for donating, Carol would pay for Molly's graduate school. Arrangements were subsequently made for Carol, Sam, and

Molly to meet with a mental health professional for an evaluation and to discuss various psychosocial aspects of the donation.

During the meeting with Carol and Sam, it became clear to the psychologist that Carol had not sufficiently grieved the loss of her fertility. Carol was supported by Sam in her determination to have her niece as an egg donor. Both seemed unwilling to consider any suggestion that Molly could, for any number of reasons, potentially be an inappropriate donor. They insisted that Molly be "evaluated" as soon as possible so that the donation procedure could move quickly. The couple added that they did not plan to tell the potential offspring about having been created through ovum donation by a family member. They saw no point in doing so since the child would simply be a part of the family gene pool in any case. They indicated that they had full confidence in Molly and the other members of the family that the "secret" would not be revealed.

The meeting with Molly was also revealing. Molly indicated that she had had a past history of depression—one bout of depression followed an elective abortion during her junior year of college. Molly also confessed that she felt overwhelmed when she heard about the injections, medications, and time commitment involved in the medical procedure. She became tearful when she realized that her first genetic offspring would actually belong to someone else. Nonetheless, she seemed determined to proceed because, "In the long run, this will pay off for everyone." She added that she and her mother both felt very sorry for Carol and Sam. During the interview with the psychologist, Molly was told that, if she did not wish to be a donor to her aunt and uncle, the psychologist would protect her from potential anger and resentment from her relatives. Molly shook her head and said that it did not matter because having graduate school paid for was "worth the trouble."

The mental health professional in this case reported orally and in a written report to the physician and staff that coercion, both overt and covert, appeared to be a key factor in this case. The generational difference between aunt and niece also contributed to the coercive aspect of the arrangement. The clinician stressed that to move forward with the donation under such circumstances could have short- and long-term negative effects on the family, including the potential offspring. The physician, being pressured by

Carol and Sam, decided to move ahead, despite the psychological report.

One day following the egg retrieval, Molly's mother contacted the physician to say that she and her sister were at odds about disclosure to others about the donation. Carol's sister essentially felt that it was important that Molly share details of the donation with friends and other family members. Her mother noted, "Molly has done a wonderful thing for Carol and Sam, and others should know about it." The physician, in turn, contacted the mental health professional to ask that an intervention be made as soon as possible. The embryos would have to be transferred soon, and some resolution was necessary,

The mental health clinician in this instance again felt angry and resentful about being "used' in this fashion. In this case, her clinical judgment and opinion had been overruled, and she was being asked to "fix" an untenable situation in a matter of hours. Her anger and indignation were aimed not only at the patients and family members, but also at the physician. Taking a neutral, supportive stance in this case was impossible. However, it appeared that the emotional needs and psychological status of the 21-year-old donor should take priority. The clinician met with Molly and later with Carol and Sam. Molly was tearful and stated that the medications were making her "emotional" and "sad." It also appeared to the therapist that the donation process rekindled feelings of loss surrounding her earlier abortion. Molly stated that she wanted to talk with her friends about what was going on. Carol and Sam were indignant and felt that Molly should just "give it some time, and move on." They stated that their privacy and personal decisions were of utmost importance.

Although the mental health professional felt an increasing dislike for Carol and Sam, she ultimately tried to be supportive of all parties. Her recommendation was to freeze all the embryos until the crisis could be resolved in some way. The therapist clearly saw Molly as her primary patient, and her emotional well-being was a critical factor. Despite her negative feelings and outrage in having been pulled into this chaotic situation, the clinician felt that she had been consistently true to herself and her professional judgment. Ultimately, Molly became an ongoing psychotherapy patient. The embryos are still frozen and no decision has been made regarding their future use. Carol and Sam were referred to another therapist in an effort to help them resolve their fertility issues and general feelings about ovum donation.

CONCLUSION

The fast-growing and ever-changing field of reproductive medicine presents unusual challenges for mental health professionals. It seems that therapists must often come face to face with their own personal biases, values, and beliefs about this technology and what it can or should offer to patients. These feelings and views, in turn, can affect the treatment process in both positive and negative ways. If a therapist is aware of his or her value system or negative feelings about various treatments, the easier it will be to say no to being involved in an arrangement that is clinically inappropriate or unethical.

Therapists' own past experiences will also affect their preconceptions about some of the treatments that are requested by patients and agreed to by medical professionals. It is not uncommon, for example, for psychotherapists working in reproductive medicine to have had some personal experience with infertility. Their personal feelings about treatment and various family-building alternatives may sometimes cloud their clinical judgment when working with certain patients.

It is critical that mental health professionals working in the field of infertility and reproductive technology keep in mind that negative preconceptions or countertransference can be important and helpful sources of clinical information. A good psychotherapist is allowed to have negative feelings about patients or the circumstances in which they are involved. How these feelings are acknowledged and dealt with, however, will be critical in the treatment or "nontreatment" of a patient. Understanding and accepting the negative countertransference and negative preconceptions will ultimately allow the mental health clinician to be true to him- or herself. In so doing, he or she can also be genuine and true to the patient. It is hoped, too, that the mental health professional will, in the long run, help set standards of appropriate and ethical judgment regarding what types of treatment options infertility clinics should consider for their clientele.

5

THERAPIST ANGER, DESPAIR, CYNICISM

Judith Kottick

*P*rofessionals must keep in mind that, unlike most other medical specialties, the infertility field has an obvious and unique component; treatment affects not only the "patient," that is, the would-be parents, but an important third party as well—the child. Because of this need to balance the competing emotional interests of the different parties, for the mental health professional working on the team there are occasions of personal and professional conflict. It is possible that, despite diligent work to protect the interests of one party, the interests of others have been neglected. While it is true that reproductive freedom in our society allows the fertile world to conceive a child whether or not it is beneficial to the individual, the child, or society, for this fertile majority there are no complicit professionals assisting in the event.

In their role as team members in "aiding and abetting" in the treatment of infertility, clinicians are faced with a range of emotions and existential issues, with barely a roadmap for guidance. Yes, there are excellent governing bodies that propose various standards for medical practice, and there are subcommittees that look at specific ethical concerns. However, these guidelines do not delve into the deep emotional impact faced by front-line workers, nor can they possibly contemplate every aspect of a situation that might arise. It takes the amazing creativity of an infertility patient to do that!

Bear in mind that, in the overwhelming majority of cases, participating in the achievement of a pregnancy can be quite a heady experience. And when the pregnancy attempt fails, clinicians and support staff who have become connected to these patients may confront their own sadness, sense of failure, and, if you will, impotence. The collective teamwork that is involved in this process has the potential both to pull the staff together as a cohesive unit, all working toward the same end, or to pit them against each other as they battle turf issues, power struggles, ethical disagreements, their sense of impotence, and the everyday pressures of working with an emotional patient population.

The team in a reproductive medical practice generally consists of physicians, nurses, embryologists, lab technicians, support staff such as office workers and clinical assistants, and a mental health professional. In this context, the psychologist or social worker is generally not called on to do long-term psychotherapy or necessarily to help the patient with ingrained, unresolved conflicts. More often, the patient is looking for emotional support, strategies for making treatment decisions, relief from the depression and anxiety that come with the territory, stress reduction, assistance with couple issues that arise, and education about third-party reproduction. Generally, the standard of care in the industry would make counseling available but not mandatory for all patients except for those participating in third party reproduction, who are required to attend one counseling session. Third-party reproduction counseling includes recipients of donor gametes, egg donors, both known or anonymous, known sperm donors, surrogates or gestational carriers, and the intended parents. Anonymous sperm donors fall under the domain of a sperm bank. In actuality, programs vary widely in their treatment of the psychological component of infertility; some have no affiliated mental health professional and no mandatory counseling at all; others require all IVF patients to consult with a counselor.

During my seven years as a clinical social worker on the staff of a thriving infertility program, I observed and became embroiled in the highly charged atmosphere of the creation of life. Although the physician frequently has the least physical contact with the patient, save the embryologist, he or she is most often responsible for making the majority of the decisions regarding the patient's treatment. For the physician, there is generally a drive to succeed in treating the infertility, as well there should be, but this can be accomplished (or not) at great cost to the patient ethically, financially, physically, or emotionally.

This scenario often puts the goals of the medical staff at cross purposes with those of the psychologist or social worker, who, as he or she is trained to do, takes a broader view of the situation than simply the treatment of a physical ailment. There are complicated societal issues at stake, and, because the field is largely unregulated, individual programs are left to make their own decisions regarding treatment criteria—which particular procedure to recommend, or whether to treat at all. For the mental health professional, wrestling with the ethical predicament of treatment criteria not only creates personal and professional conflict, but also can create havoc within the team as well. Thus, the question for the infertility counselor is this: whose side are you on—that of the patient, a third party (i.e., an egg donor or surrogate), the unborn child, or the infertility clinic?

Consider the case of Allie and Beth, two sisters from a large Hispanic family, who with their spouses sought infertility treatment together. Allie and her husband, Clark, had a previous course of infertility care and became pregnant on their fourth in vitro fertilization attempt. In her eighth month, however, Allie delivered a stillborn and developed a raging infection, putting her own life at risk. Several months later, Allie and Clark returned to the clinic to utilize cryopreserved embryos but did not become pregnant.

In the meantime, Beth and her husband, Dave, were also experiencing infertility and did their own IVF cycle. With no fertilized embryos resulting from the attempt, Beth was referred for ovum donation with the diagnosis of ovarian failure. At this point, as close sisters, Allie and Beth realized they could both benefit from Allie's ability to produce viable eggs. They wanted to share Allie's eggs by splitting them between the two sisters. On the face of it, from the medical standpoint, there were no issues, since donation between sisters has been standard protocol for years.

The implications were troubling, however, when this case was considered from a psychological point of view. The most obvious concern was the possibility that Beth would become pregnant with the help of her sister's eggs, while Allie would not. During the consultation, it became clear, not surprisingly, that Allie and Clark were still in the throes of grief from the loss of their baby less than a year earlier. The desire to protect Allie and Clark from further heartache was enormous. How would they cope with the possibility of being responsible for the birth of a niece or nephew, while childless themselves? Would they wonder if they had cheated themselves by giving up the "good eggs"? What if they were never successful? How would failure affect the sisters' relationship; surely there would be enormous feelings of guilt on Beth's part? How would this complex family situation affect the child? Alternatively, what if the hoped-for scenario did work for both of them. Would the children be caught up in a web of competition or comparisons? What, if anything, would they be told about their conception and family relationships?

This case illustrates the challenges and ambiguity of the world of reproductive medicine. Here is the chance to help two stable and loving couples achieve parenthood, through a procedure that is medically routine and financially beneficial for the medical practice. There is certainly no coercion going on, as the patients are asking, if not begging, for the procedure. But there is a risk of harming the primary patients, Allie and Clark, who are still grieving for their lost child, as well as the family system as a whole, including the potential child or children.

In this case, mine was the only dissenting opinion to moving forward as Allie and Beth desired. I suggested the alternative plan of giving Allie and Clark the opportunity to have a baby first before helping Beth. This proved an unpopular approach, as Beth and Dave were unwilling to wait what could be years finally to become parents. Moreover, the physicians were not willing to deny the patients' request on the *chance* that psychological problems might develop. I ended up in the unenviable position of attempting to defend a stance that angered everyone involved. As Allie and Beth prepared to move through their cycle, I experienced a mixture of emotions. Although I felt defeated that my opinion had been overridden, I also wanted to support these two hopeful couples. I wished that human behavior were as clear-cut as science and medicine.

In her novel *The Secret*, Eva Hoffman (2002) explores the psychological ramifications of living life as an individual created through the advances of technology. The protagonist, a young woman who searches for her identity, confronts the scientist who helped give her life:

> "You never thought about me, did you?" I said quickly, "You never thought what it would be like for me."
> "Why . . ." he said again, looking baffled, "It was what your mother wanted. We did it with your mother's full consent."
> "But what about me?" I said. "Didn't anybody think, didn't anybody imagine what it would be like to be me?" [p. 98].

It is exactly this question that is in the purview of the infertility counselor, and, when I am thinking about the feelings of the unborn child, often dominates my late-night thoughts. We have to wonder, at what point is it better for a child not to be born? While there exist "wrongful birth" and "wrongful life" legal proceedings, these pertain to physical defects or injury, and not to psychological harm (Strong, 1996).

Although the medical procedures are often relatively simple, the emotional conflicts are complex, nuanced and multilayered. Fran, a 24-year-old single woman who lived with her parents, sought assistance in becoming pregnant by donor sperm. As part of the routine testing and screening procedures for patients using donor gametes, Fran, an attractive, blue-eyed blond, was sent for a counseling session. During her visit, Fran reported that she had never been in a serious romantic relationship and was still a virgin. She had always lived with her parents. She was not experienced with gynecological exams and had anxiety about the upcoming routine medical tests, such as the vaginal ultrasounds, saline sonogram, and hysterosalpingogram. Despite her fears, however, she was willing to be subjected to any procedure in her quest to have a child.

When questioned about her urgency, Fran reported that her mother had experienced infertility for 10 years before she eventually conceived without medical intervention. Subsequently, she was unable to have more children, despite her longing to do so. Fran feared that she, too, might be infertile, and becoming a mother was more important to her than being involved in a relationship. She was always aware that her parents wanted another child, and she was dissatisfied with being an only child. In fact, given that she worked full time, Fran envisioned her parents providing child care for their grandchild. I wondered, was this a child for Fran, or a wish to please her parents and provide the longed-for child/sibling for her family? Despite the invitation to explore her motivations more thoroughly with additional counseling sessions, Fran was not interested. Along with the invasive medical testing she agreed to, Fran was willing to fulfill her counseling requirement but would go no further.

When Fran left her session, I felt unsettled. Many concerns loomed in my mind. From an ethical viewpoint, we are separating reproduction and sex to the point where it is no longer necessary to be a sexual being in order to bear children. Additionally, considering the case from a psychological point of view, I was deeply troubled by the enmeshed and incestuous overtones of the family's dynamics. The nurse who worked closely with Fran observed that Fran's father seemed overly involved, acting at times like the "partner." He took messages regarding medications, insisted on mixing all drugs, and gave the injections to his daughter. How much should we make of these emotionally incestuous behaviors? It is an unusual scenario for a young woman in her 20s, still living with and, at the very least, emotionally dependent on her parents, to be so desperate to have a child that she would prefer to undergo expensive, uncomfortable, and invasive procedures rather than looking for a loving relationship and parenting partner. Fran was not infertile.

Of course, with increasing frequency, there are many single women who have not found partners and who decide to pursue single parenthood. But, according to Jacob (1999), studies have shown that single women electing to be single mothers tend to be independent, financially secure, and highly thoughtful for several years before making this decision. This was not the case for Fran. I recommended postponing fertility treatment to give Fran the opportunity to explore more fully her urgent desire to become pregnant since no fertility issues were detected. Although the outcome for a child conceived in such a situation might include issues that would keep a family therapist busy, I felt that the most pressing concern was the nature of Fran's relationship with her father.

However, the medical program did not mandate ongoing psychological counseling and, in the absence of concrete data, would not go against Fran's wishes. The program's decision left me in a quandary. I felt stymied by the physicians' refusal to consider psychological care as an essential component of infertility treatment. Would they ignore a fibroid in the uterus if they felt it might "infect" the developing fetus, even if the patient wanted them to do so? On the other hand, I struggled with the notion that Fran was an adult who was not asking for my approval or even my opinion.

There is controversy in the mental health field about whether or not "gatekeeping" is within the purview of counselors working in the realm of reproductive medicine. Several views are in evidence. Some professionals believe they are advocates of the child; others are unwilling to take the ultimate step of deciding who can or cannot parent; and a third group "tend to exclude from treatment only those couples in extreme situations" (Cooper, 1997, p. 44). While the gatekeeping role is expected for social workers in the field of adoption, it is by no means mandated in the domain of reproductive medicine.

In our country, reproductive freedom exists for the fertile world, regardless of their fitness as parents. Do we have a right to impose higher standards for those people who are infertile (Cooper, 1997)? If not for our knowledge of the potentially destructive forces that lurk beneath a family's surface and compromise a child's ability to thrive, the gatekeeping issue would not be so compelling. We certainly assume that our right to autonomy allows us, as human beings, the freedom to make our own choices (within the legal boundaries of our society), to carry on our lives, reproduction (and in some cases, death) as we see fit. As long as we give informed consent to legal medical procedures, we feel that we are entitled to them. But when a procedure has the potential to affect another human being, the standard is less clear . . . Or is it?

Connell (1990) explores the issues of government regulation in reproductive medicine and points out that favoring an unborn child's rights may potentially compromise the rights of people who want to become parents. Therefore, "To ensure people the broadest scope of reproductive freedom, only regulations actually proved to protect the fetus or child, without materially restricting the persons attempting to procreate, should be sustained" (pp. 72–73). Lantos (1990) considers this "divided loyalty" concept to be one in which the therapist has to reckon with the potentially divergent interests of the would-be parents, the offspring, and the larger community. He likens the issue to one confronted by obstetricians: "Psychiatrists who weigh the best interest of the child above the desires of the parents will enter the ethical thicket of maternal–fetal conflicts" (p. 91). In other words, physicians are sometimes called on to choose a treatment that is beneficial to the child while increasing potential harm to the mother. There are times, he concludes, when the child's welfare takes precedence over the parents' (p. 91). Warnock (2002) looks at inclusion and exclusion criteria for infertility treatment. She argues that, although there may be individual cases that challenge our moral and ethical sensibilities, it would be difficult to impose a strict set of standards based on moral grounds that would govern who receives treatment. Once we start down that path, she reasons, how far would we go? Would eugenics be far behind?

We must accept the possibility that some children born through reproductive technology may not be parented optimally and may, in fact, be parented poorly. But the ultimate responsibility "must lie, as it always does, with the parents of those children; and if they fail in their duty, then as is regularly the case, society must take over" (p. 53). Alternatively, Robertson and Crockin (1996) support the case for paying attention to the potential child's welfare and advise that "programs should be run and structured to minimize harm to offspring" (p. 154). Mahowald (1996) also advocates considering a child's well-being in determining whether or not treatment is appropriate. She quotes a physician from Michigan who reasons that, even though fertile people do not have to prove their competence as potential parents, "'I am responsible only for that over which I have some control'" (p. 264).

In the absence of consensus on the welfare of the child question, it appears to be "every man for himself" in determining how each program considers this issue. There are no guidelines set out by the American Society for Reproductive Medicine (ASRM). Widely disparate but rarely agreed upon views on the matter govern standards regarding the not-yet-conceived child. To complicate the situation even further, there is yet another person to think about when third-party reproduction is involved. If a gamete donor or surrogate is in the picture, how much weight is given to the "right" (or maybe it is simply an expectation) to assist in bringing a child into the world who will be parented, at the very least, adequately? Another case example may help to illuminate this point.

Gail, in her mid-40s and with a 52-year-old husband, was previously treated at another infertility program in California. In her initial counseling session with me, Gail revealed that, after several years of treatment and IVF, she finally became pregnant. Although this pregnancy was initially heralded with great joy, the situation quickly turned to despair when Gail developed hyperemesis gravidarum, a condition of severe morning sickness resulting in excessive vomiting, which for some women can be debilitating and may result in dehydration and hospitalization. As the pregnancy progressed, the fetus developed normally, but Gail became increasingly emotionally unstable as she reacted to the unending nausea and vomiting. Within a couple of months, she was unable to bear this condition and asked to terminate the pregnancy. Physicians and her husband attempted to talk her out of this drastic measure, but she found the physical discomfort so intolerable that she insisted on proceeding with an abortion.

Shortly thereafter, she experienced remorse and regret and began trying to conceive again through IVF. She became more and more demanding and abusive to the staff as she was unsuccessful in subsequent attempts, and she was encouraged to seek treatment at another program. With IVF using her own eggs no longer an option due to advancing age, she decided, reluctantly, to pursue egg donation at our program. During her routine donor egg recipient interview, the above scenario was laid out to me, and we began to explore the possibility that a future pregnancy could result in the very same hyperemesis situation. What would she do in this case? According to Gail, she would be prepared this time and would have the perspective to understand that she is "out of her mind" when in this condition. She believed she would be able to withstand the discomfort and also felt that she could not endure the regret she would experience with another termination, compounded by her first loss.

As the treatment progressed, Gail became angry, demanding, and verbally abusive to the staff. She managed to pit one nurse against another; she saw one as a savior and the other as conspiring against her. She had the entire staff questioning each other, in addition to questioning Gail's potential fitness as a parent. Although Gail's behavior was probably outside the norm, even for the typically emotional fertility patient, her attempt to seize control wherever possible could also be understood as a consequence of the trauma suffered from her previous pregnancy. Her abuse toward the staff could be interpreted as a defense against enormous guilt and anxiety. As is often the case, it was difficult to discern the degree to which her current behavior was predictive of her emotional state when, and if, she were to become a parent. But the question still remained: would she be able to carry out another pregnancy in the event of hyperemesis, and, further, was this a matter even relevant to those of us who would be providing the means to a pregnancy, if, indeed, we are not meant to be gatekeepers?

To complicate the case further, Gail recruited her own ovum donor through an advertisement. She met her but they were not on close, personal terms. The donor was lovely and met the ovum donor screening criteria as set forth by ASRM guidelines. However, as Gail tried to micromanage the donor's cycle, this young woman began to get wind of Gail's erratic behavior and started to question whether she should be involved as a donor at all. Aside from the issue of the degree to which nonfamily donors and recipients should have contact, a controversial subject in itself, Gail's case also brought up another quandary: What is our responsibility to the gamete donor? What are his or her "rights" when there is the chance that the pregnancy will be terminated, and if it is not, that the recipient may not be an optimal parent?

In most anonymous gamete donor programs on the East Coast, it is typical for recipients to have varying amounts of nonidentifying information about the ovum or sperm donor to help provide a sense of connection and physical match to the donor. The recipients may receive information about ethnicity, eye and hair color, and the medical histories of the young women and men (by way of sperm bank) as well as their immediate and extended family members. Some programs also give information about the donors' personality traits, SAT scores, hobbies, interests, and the colleges attended. On the other hand, the donors receive no information whatsoever about the recipients and often have no idea if a successful pregnancy has even occurred.

This scenario is very different from the current trend in domestic adoption, where the birth parents have extensive information about potential adoptive parents and can choose the family where their child will be placed. Certainly, gamete donation and adoption are different entities; the philosophy for donors is that they should be able to separate from their gametes and *not* see the egg or sperm as a child; whereas, for the birth mother, the child is a living, breathing human being.

I often wonder, does this mean we have no responsibility to meet the donor's expectations? Is the donor really better off in the dark? It may be the counselor's job during the screening process to highlight for the donor the fact that recipients are not psychologically screened in the same way that donors are. Even so, it is probably safe to say that, for many donors, the financial incentive overrides their curiosity about the recipients. However, this does not detract from the fact that many altruistic and idealistic young women anonymously donate their eggs in good faith, expecting the recipients to be the type of parents they would want themselves.

Although there is scant research on the expectations of gamete donors, and even less on the aftereffects of donating, I did speak with a young woman who works as a nurse with donors and recipients in an infertility program and who had been an egg donor herself while in college, before marriage and children. Working with recipients, she admitted, had "ruined" her experience of being a donor. She had been unprepared for the types of behavior she would encounter in the patients and worried where her eggs had ended up. After having her own children, she said, her concern became even more salient. This is a perspective few donors have, but it does point to an important party whose interests might be considered (but what to degree?), along with those of the recipient couples and the potential children. In Gail's case, the limited contact she had with her donor was enough to give her pause and question the advisability of moving forward. Yet she did follow through, and the question remained for me, would she have done so had she known all the facts?

I was left to ponder these questions in my assigned role, which might be described as psychoeducator. The role does not encourage any in-depth analysis of the appropriateness of medical treatment, or what the physicians might deem "fortune telling." At the same time, in Gail's case I was compelled to perform another role, not atypical in this setting, that of mediator. The staff became angry at each other, owing to Gail's successful efforts to split the nurses and support personnel between "good" and "bad." Even those who were deemed good were furious at Gail's behavior, and no one wanted to talk to her. As the staff became less responsive, Gail's acting-out behavior increased and a unanimous chorus of "Help!" came my way.

I quickly discovered that acting as a source of support for team members was an important part of my position, as was the role of disciplinarian (i.e., letting the patient know that abusive behavior toward the employees is unacceptable). With this in mind, I encouraged the staff to view Gail more sympathetically. I helped them identify with her losses, educated them on the fine points of "splitting" in hopes they would stop viewing each other as adversaries, and set limits with Gail so she would stop interfering with her donor's cycle and to prevent her harsh behavior with my colleagues from creating further conflict. These actions would all have seemed worthwhile except that I had qualms about whether or not this case should move forward in the first place. However, it was not my decision.

In these clinical illustrations I have highlighted examples of situations that raised doubts in my mind as to the advisability of the use of reproductive technology. In these cases, my concerns were generally overlooked in favor of the patients' desire for treatment. I was not necessarily in favor of denying treatment to these individuals and couples (although in some cases I might have been), but I would have desired a debate and an ethical framework within which to make decisions. In some programs, there are ethics committees prepared to deal with these types of cases. I imagine that a decision made after a thoughtful process, in which numerous points of view are given equal weight, and a consensus, or semblance thereof, is reached, might seem like a decision of substance. In the absence of this experience, many mental health providers are left feeling ineffectual and trivial, while raising the question of whether decisions are made based on ethics or economics.

While the cases presented so far have illuminated instances that undervalued the mental health perspective, there are times when, alternatively, the authority invested in the role seems like too much responsibility. In my experience, these situations generally involve donor egg and gestational surrogacy evaluations. The young women who present themselves for these evaluations are usually medically appropriate for the "job," but it is the psychological component that is less clear-cut. We, as mental health evaluators, do our best with a time-limited clinical interview and crude psychological tests to make judgments of the fitness of the candidates for these services. But, with little objective data to base decisions on and virtually no long-term studies, it is an inexact process, at best.

In addition, the women who apply for these roles are motivated to present themselves in a positive light and may withhold important information that they feel might disqualify them. The candidates know that they are just that—potential donors or gestational carriers who may not be accepted for these roles. However, if it is possible to speculate that there is a narcissistic component to a woman's belief that her genetic material or womb would be a desired entity, rejection may be suffered as a serious narcissistic injury. What does it say to a candidate if that which defines her identity as a woman is not desired? Proficient as we are in the mental health field at developing a relationship with a person, making him or her feel safe and drawing out the truth, in this role we are free to use this newly formed relationship to decide against accepting the very person who has offered to perform a generous act, whether he or she is financially motivated or otherwise.

In these instances, I have felt deceptive and manipulative, gaining a candidate's trust, only to use the information "against" her. This is very different from a job interview, where an offer is made (or not) based on objective criteria about ability and experience. In the case of donor and gestational carrier evaluations, although we believe, and it could be true, that we are protecting people (both the candidate herself and the recipients/intended parents) by excluding them from the process, it does not negate the possibility that a woman may leave the screening process worse off than when she came in. I feel a sense of responsibility to these women, especially in a case where the strength of the woman's candidacy is not straightforward.

Another case example may illustrate this point. Helen was a 34-year-old gestational carrier candidate who was divorced and raising five children on her own. The children ranged in age from one to 16 years old. Her ex-husband was only minimally involved and provided no financial support. She did not have family nearby and worked full time three long days a week. These bare facts alone might be reason enough for Helen to be rejected, as one might assume that she is burdened enough in her life without adding the unknown course of a pregnancy. In the best-case scenario, if there were no complications, just by virtue of being pregnant and participating in this process, Helen might take attention away from her own children or be unable to attend to this very coveted pregnancy in the manner the intended parents might demand.

However, Helen presented herself as an admirable woman, one of those very capable people who has her priorities straight and has managed work and child care to her best advantage. She obviously loved and cherished her children, and, on top of it all, appeared emotionally stable and likeable. Her psychological test results were completely within normal limits. Despite my doubts about her appropriateness "on paper," I was drawn to Helen and found myself thinking that she might be an acceptable candidate. There was also information that Helen had been exceedingly responsible and proactive during the prescreening process, which always gives useful data about how responsive a candidate will be to the unending details and inconveniences that will dog her during the year or so she is involved as a gestational carrier.

Making the decision more difficult, the intended parents who had been matched with Helen had started to develop a positive relationship with her and were applying pressure to have her approved. I was also influenced by the reality that the financial gain from this experience could greatly enhance Helen's life. Although we try to rule out financial coercion as motivation for women "volunteering" for this activity, there is no question that monetary gain is an incentive for many people who participate as donors and carriers. Like many fellow gestational carrier prospects, Helen verbalized both financial and altruistic reasons for wanting to participate. I reasoned, if everything were to go smoothly, this arrangement would probably be fine, and two families would gain immeasurably.

What could not be predicted, though, was the risk and effect of potential complications. I worried, what if Helen ended up on restricted activity or bed rest, if she felt sick or incapacitated, had a difficult delivery requiring longer term recuperation, or experienced any of the myriad problems that could arise? She had a limited support system and did free-lance work with no job security or benefits. Her five young children depended solely on her, so that any ensuing complications could adversely affect all her children as well as her pregnancy and the developing baby. Pregnancy had been uneventful and easy for Helen in the past, and she was pregnant with four children in tow only a year before.

Ultimately, though, I could not justify placing Helen or the intended parents in the position of potentially coping with a problem that could put Helen and her family, or the fetus, into a state of crisis, even if the risk was unlikely. Yet, as the person with the authority to make this decision, I wanted to give Helen this opportunity rather than deprive her of an experience that could be highly rewarding on many levels (as it is for most carriers). Additionally, I wanted to respect the intended parents' desire to achieve their long awaited goal in a timely manner, by sanctioning this arrangement. In my decision to reject Helen, I felt professionally responsible and personally conflicted.

Little did I know how complicated the issues would be when I entered into this field. The wish to assist people in detangling their unhealthy patterns, to provide a deep personal connection, and to have the opportunity to help fellow human beings improve their lives are some of the reasons that mental health professionals become counselors, social workers, and psychologists. There are always varying degrees of success in this endeavor. In this job, though, there are times when I have feared I might be involved in making someone's life worse. For instance, what if I help someone get pregnant and she ends up with triplets and is not equipped to handle such a task, or I watch a marriage disintegrate because one partner insists on a treatment option that to the other is intolerable. While oftentimes those of us who work in a fertility program do not have the opportunity to hear the ending of the stories we have begun, there are times when details do emerge. What follows is an example of a case, unlike those previously presented, that did not ring alarm bells at the time or leave the team worried about the future. It reminds us that, despite our concern for the patients and their potential children, we cannot predict what will happen.

As a colleague recently reminded me, we can sometimes predict future behavior on the basis of past behavior, but patients, in our brief encounters, tell us very little of the past.

Jim and Kay, a Canadian couple in their 20s, did a second IVF cycle and became pregnant with triplets, having had no pregnancy at all during their first two attempts at IVF. Appropriately concerned about the prospect of carrying and raising triplets, they requested a consultation with me to discuss multifetal reduction versus parenting triplets. During the session, they discussed their lifestyle, religious beliefs, infertility history, and, briefly, personal histories. They mentioned that they could arrange their work schedules so that they could take turns providing child care and would not need, nor could they afford, outside help.

Like others before them in this predicament, they felt unable to discuss the triplet issue with friends or family members for fear of harsh judgment for even considering a reduction procedure. The decision came down to their personal belief that they would be unable to handle triplets given their financial status and the support system available, weighed against their religious beliefs, which would oppose the termination of a fetus. Jim and Kay were thoughtful and respectful of each other while working through this dilemma and appeared equally present and emotionally invested in finding a solution they could live with. In the end, though sad and concerned about their spiritual "status," they decided to reduce to a twin pregnancy, with the goal of a sane and healthy life for their children and themselves. Several months after seeing them, I spoke to both Jim and Kay on the phone to follow up on our meeting. They had undergone the reduction procedure and primarily expressed relief, with some lingering guilt feelings. Overall, they were excited about the pregnancy and the impending birth and felt they had made the best decision, given their circumstances.

Eighteen months later, I received a telephone call from a social worker in their hospital's pediatric department. Jim and Kay had appeared with their young son and daughter, both of whom presented with subdural hematomas, defined on the Medline Health Information website as a "collection of blood on the surface of the brain" (Medline, 2002a). Physicians were baffled as to the cause of this condition. The symptoms were consistent with those of shaken baby syndrome (Medline, 2002b), but the parents and maternal grandmother, the only caregivers, vigorously denied any such behavior. Shaken baby syndrome is a "severe form of head injury caused by violently shaking an infant or child. . . . An angry parent or caregiver may shake a baby to punish or quiet him or her. Many times they do not intend to harm the baby."

The social worker who called wanted me to know that hospital officials were looking for any information that might help them with their investigation. Other medical explanations were explored, but the fact that the babies had identical injuries made shaken baby syndrome their leading hypothesis.

As I think back to my contact with Jim and Kay a year and a half earlier, I cannot imagine they would be implicated in such a scenario. I assumed there must be another explanation. Meanwhile, the babies had surgery to drain excess fluid from the brain, and, during the couple of weeks of hospitalization, investigations continued. Finally, after weeks of denial, Jim, in an emotional confession, admitted that he had, in fact, shaken his son and daughter in a moment of parental despair. Kay, apparently, did not know he had done so.

Whether or not there were indications in Jim's past that could have predicted this behavior, I do not know. Many parents admit to fantasies of shaking their babies, or worse, to stop incessant crying, but most control the impulse. I wished I had explored Jim and Kay's family histories more fully. In this setting, though, the majority of patients are not requesting psychotherapy; they expect instead a specific problem or decision to be resolved in a session or two. Ideally, we can inspire those who are really struggling to seek therapy and enjoy the benefits of longer term counseling. However, part of the frustration of this job is accepting the limitations of the role and living with uncertainty about the future.

In the same way that I did not anticipate what would transpire in the previous case, I could not imagine the fate of Allie and Clark, Beth and Dave, Fran, or Gail. As it turns out, we have heard from most of them over the years, and the news appears good, at least on the surface. Allie and Beth both became pregnant, Allie with a singleton and Beth with twins. In yearly holiday cards, they express heartfelt appreciation to our team for helping them to create their two wonderful families. Gail came back several years after her daughter was born to talk about the disposition of her frozen embryos. She told us that she had, in fact, had a difficult pregnancy with severe nausea and vomiting but was able to hold on until the end. She brought her daughter to the office; she was a delightful and exceptionally precocious toddler. We observed that Gail was overbearing as a mother but certainly adoring and nurturing. Fran also became pregnant, but the outcome remains a mystery. Naturally, these families, like all families, will have issues to contend with down the line, and it is possible that the initial concerns, or other related issues, will become relevant in time. Still, it is a sobering lesson in the limits of my role as a clinical social worker in a reproductive medicine practice.

What has become clear to me is that, for the privilege of helping people build their families as part of a multidisciplinary team, I must also be prepared to withstand the sense of discomfort, frustration, and confusion that accompanies the task. At times I am forced to struggle with points of view that challenge my personal or professional beliefs. I grapple with the degree to which I am accountable for decisions made by other professionals on the team that I feel are emotionally or ethically questionable. I wonder whether I am being "judgmental" or "ethically responsible" when I disagree with certain procedures. I question how to weigh a person's right to make choices regarding infertility treatment against my educated perspective on human behavior and concern for the unborn child. Along with my colleagues, I have learned to live with uncertainty, to confront the implications of new technology, and to think seriously about futuristic issues that many people consider only in their wildest dreams or nightmares. So far, it is an emotional challenge I am willing to take.

REFERENCES

Connell, C. K. (1990), Legal implications of the new reproductive technologies. In: *Psychiatric Aspects of Reproductive Technology*, ed. N. L. Stotland. Washington, DC: American Psychiatric Press, pp. 67–85.

Cooper, S. (1997), Ethical issues associated with the new reproductive technologies. In: *Infertility: Psychological Issues and Counseling Strategies*, ed. S. R. Leiblum. New York: Wiley, pp. 41–66.

Covington, S. N. (1995), The role of the mental health professional in reproductive medicine. *Fertil. & Steril.*, 64:895–897.

Hoffman, E. (2002), *The Secret.* New York: Public Affairs.

Jacob, M. C. (1999), Lesbian couples and single women. In: *Infertility Counseling: A Comprehensive Handbook for Clinicians*, ed. L. H. Burns & S. N. Covington. New York: Parthenon, pp. 267–281.

Lantos, J. D. (1990), Second-generation ethical issues in the new reproductive technology: Divided loyalty, indications, and the research agenda. In: *Psychiatric Aspects of Reproductive Technology*, ed. N. L. Stotland. Washington, DC: American Psychiatric Press, pp. 87–96.

Mahowald, M. M. (1996), Conceptual and ethical considerations in medically assisted reproduction. In: *Family Building Through Egg and Sperm Donation: Medical, Legal, and Ethical Issues*, ed. M. M. Seibel & S. L. Crockin. Sudbury, MA: Jones & Bartlett, pp. 262–273.

Medline (2002a), Subdural hematoma. http://www.nlm.nih.gov/medlineplus/ency/article/000713.html.

———(2002b), Shaken baby syndrome. http://www.nlm.nih.gov/medlineplus/ency/article/000004.html.

Robertson, J. A. & Crockin, S. L. (1996), Legal issues in egg donation. In: *Family Building Through Egg and Sperm Donation: Medical, Legal, and Ethical Issues*, ed. M. M. Seibel & S. L. Crockin. Sudbury, MA: Jones & Bartlett, pp. 144–157.

Strong, C. (1996), Genetic screening in oocyte donation: Ethical and legal aspects. In: *New Ways of Making Babies*, ed. C. Cohen. Bloomington: Indiana University Press, pp. 122–137.

Warnock, M. (2002), *Making Babies.* Oxford: Oxford University Press.

6

RIDING THE ELEPHANT IN THE ROOM

How I Use Countertransference in Couples Therapy

Todd Essig

*I*t's built in, a "design feature." A couple comes regularly to your office. You engage them in the most helpful way you know how as dictated by your professional training and experience and by the person you are. You listen, respond, and act. But then, as treatment progresses, you begin to notice thoughts, feelings, physical sensations, and the like. They are just there. Even though safely ensconced in your professional identity, this basic fact of your humanity remains; you are a person engaged with other people and you will have your own experiences.

These private experiences are simply human inevitabilities built into the interactional structure of our complex therapeutic relationships. And these inevitabilities lead to the key questions motivating this chapter: what to do about or with these personal, private experiences? Should you embrace them? Try to ignore them? Are you embarrassed by them? Do you think of them as relevant? Irrelevant? In other words, countertransference, a technical name for all those personal, private experiences therapists have in response to patients, is part of all therapeutic encounters; the questions are whether or not to use it and if so, how?

The answer I present throughout this chapter is that using countertransference can be of significant value for couples therapy. I believe our countertransference experiences can be made into clinical "gold" when we take them to be simultaneously data and puzzle. Rather than acting directly on these experiences because of a naïve faith in their value or, at the other extreme, trying to ignore them out of a belief that they are simply noise or indications of one's own personal problems, the approach presented here takes countertransference to be an experience to think with that is of considerable potential value. As I illustrate in the clinical material presented later, the potential clinical value of countertransference is present even when it includes powerful, destabilizing, or unpleasant thoughts, feelings, and self-states. Using reflection in a search for clinical value (i.e., riding the elephant in the room) is possible even when the experience feels like a threat to one's effective therapeutic functioning. In fact, reflectively engaging those difficult experiences often yields the most interesting results.

Thinking with countertransference is an active, ongoing process that is a routine part of clinical listening and action. We think with and not just about countertransference because we are simultaneously always in it when we are thinking about it. It is always with us. One form that thinking with countertransference can take which I have found especially useful in my work is to wonder about what is not taking place. Along with many other psychoanalysts in the interpersonal tradition (for an overview, see Lionells et al., 1995), I have come to appreciate that the gaps and omissions in experience, narration, action, and interaction are often what turn out to be of clinical significance. The clinical significance of what is not going on is seen both in the experience of the persons involved and in the system of marital interactions in which they are embedded and that which they constitute. In terms of what is not going on, couples often get into trouble when the individuals selectively inattend by not noticing what needs to be seen and when as a dyad they selectively nonparticipate by not doing to and with each other what needs to be done.

A central theme in this chapter is that the attuned therapist's countertransference is often where these inattentions and nonparticipations first register. Reflective attention paid to countertransference creates possibilities for them to be thought with and turned into valuable clinical events (Brown, 1993; Bromberg, 1998). It is in the shifting currents of our own thoughts, feelings, and self-states that previously unknown processes of selective inattention and selective nonparticipation often first appear. By thinking with these experiences, we can often formulate interventions that help couples bring observation and reflection to bear on these anxiety-avoiding gaps of inattention and nonparticipation. In my work, I pay close attention to these currents and, when using them as experiences to think with, I even go as far as to self-consciously ask myself, "What's *not* going on here?" In other words, the question, "What's not going on here?" serves as an explicit theoretical/technical scaffolding on which I work; it allows me to think with and make use of those inevitable moments of countertransferential difficulty.

This approach is particularly well suited to therapy with couples experiencing infertility. I base this conclusion on its being useful to couples I see in my practice. I should note first that my practice has been almost exclusively with heterosexual couples. While I think this approach should apply equally to same-sex couples, all the couples I talk about here are heterosexual because of the referral patterns of my practice. Second, as a private practitioner unaffiliated with any specific reproductive center or organization, I work primarily with couples who need therapeutic help beyond that provided by support groups, psychoeducational programs, and what can be seen as an emerging "standard" model of infertility counseling (Meyers, Diamond et al., 1995; Meyers, Weinshel et al., 1995; Burns and Covington, 1999; Stammer, Wischmann, and Verres, 2002).

Each of the couples with whom I have worked experienced profound difficulties coping with the technologically mediated choices, consequences, and losses secondary to involvement with assisted reproductive technologies and adoption. Other clinicians with whom they had worked often referred them to me. Many were troubled couples to begin with, and the confrontation with infertility became the occasion for seeking help that was long needed. Others were those for whom the unique traumas that come from living inside the "infertility bubble" stretched them beyond their capacity to cope. A third group of couples were those who were holding their own inside the "bubble" but faced an additional trauma that brought them to treatment, such as the horrors of the World Trade Center attack, which profoundly affected my practice. Finally, there are those who had resolved their infertility, either as parents or as living child free, but who found the resolution itself to be a fertile breeding ground for subsequent marital problems.

With these couples, the expectable and clinically well-known dramatic complexity of couples therapy takes on additional dimensions of both drama and complexity. The couple and the therapist together confront many new challenges, from questions of personal morality and biomedical ethics to understanding complex reproductive technologies and procedures. Previously settled issues about gender, sexual identity, family of origin, personal worth and self-esteem, and the interplay of intimacy and autonomy become problems once again and increase in intensity when not previously settled. Infertility transforms all these patients, usually against their will, into pioneers settling new territories of reproductive relatedness. They become, to use Papp's (2000) apt phrase, "couples on the fault line." Their challenge is to find solutions to problems in living that did not exist a generation ago.

The personal, marital, family, and social systems and the cultural tools they have at hand for addressing these new technologically mediated problems in living are often, however, ill suited to the current task. They are "hand-me-downs" developed at a time when our current technologies were not even imagined. For example, family and friends do not yet have culturally sanctioned and familiar rituals of support to console a grieving couple after the final, failed IVF cycle. And the couples themselves often do not have ways to symbolize or discuss the grief they feel, if grief is even the correct name for the affect-state experienced. What often happens is that couples use some sort of psychological duct tape to jury-rig solutions to these new technologically mediated problems in living, and this "solution" only adds to the dramatic complexity with which we become involved.

Therapists who work with these couples in the way I am describing should be prepared to explore with them this uncomfortable edge of cultural change. But being a couples therapist on the edge, especially one practicing psychoanalytically informed treatment, requires a delicate balance. We, too, must make ourselves open to the destabilizing new world of emerging reproductive technologies. Yesterday's biomedical imagination has become today's everyday clinical reality, and all indications are that our collective psychological and cultural development will continue to lag significantly behind the technological for quite some time.

Our job in the face of these often destabilizing changes includes helping to balance the new with old, familiar, embodied realities. Whether it be preserving fertility in the face of medical procedures, questions of donor gametes, the possibilities of cloning that are out there on the horizon (Rosen, 2003), or even such almost taken-for-granted processes such as IVF or international adoptions facilitated by our technologically shrunken world, there is much that remains constant. An important part of our role is to help people observe and reflect on "old-fashioned" realities, such as that kids are kids and parents are people, even when they are straddling technological/psychological fault lines and pioneering new procedures for and experiences of building a family.

Discussions of therapy with couples experiencing infertility, especially when countertransference is a topic under consideration, usually involves some discussion of whether the therapist should or should not disclose her or his own reproductive history. While a full discussion of this topic is well beyond the confines of this chapter, let me briefly share a few thoughts. The prodisclosure stance is that sharing one's reproductive history leads to a feeling of being understood and thereby supports the creation of a necessary atmosphere of safety. Moreover, within limits, therapist self-disclosure leads to patient self-disclosure. Therefore, it makes sense to put one's own history out on the table.

While I am sure that full disclosure is helpful for many clinicians in many different clinical situations, it is inconsistent with the kind of couples therapy described in this chapter. Simply put, the problem is that feeling understood is not the same thing as actually being understood. There are other ways to establish the requisite atmosphere of safety, such as an expertise in the area, genuine concern, empathic understanding, modulation of destructive patterns, and fluency in biomedical problems and techniques. It is not necessary to rely on what can frequently be an illusion of understanding. Moreover, as is the case with every illusion, there are limits to the conditions under which it operates, and the kind of intensive couples therapy herein described frequently goes beyond those limits. For example, one does not want to set up a situation where a patient defensively has to avoid awareness of significant difference between his or her experience and yours because the requisite feeling of safety is built on your having had a shared experience. It is, I believe, better to build the needed atmosphere of safety by keeping faith with the effort to understand the unique, specific features of each couple combined with a thorough understanding of the reproductive issues, problems, and treatments being discussed.

SELECTIVE INATTENTION

What is selective inattention? From the perspective of interpersonal psychoanalysis, the concept of selective inattention is both simple and powerful. It is one way to understand how people come not to know about one or another reality. The reality being selectively inattended can be located in the external world of objects, events, and other people or the internal world of representations, feelings, wishes, and thoughts. Its simplicity suits it well to being part of a conceptual scaffolding on which one can work when the countertransferential going gets tough. When we are selectively inattending one or another reality, we neither experience nor engage with it as it is or as it could be. Rather, we either do not apprehend it at all, or we obscure it with opaque fencing of private meaning. Either way, knowledge that would generate unacceptable levels of anxiety in either ourselves or others with whom we are intimately connected is not experienced. Selective inattention can thus be seen to be an elegant self-protective defensive process. In fact, it plays a central role in the security operations we use to make ourselves and the people with whom we are close feel sufficiently safe, or at least to avoid feeling unacceptably unsafe.

Stern (1995), writing about its cognitive and linguistic aspects, states, "Selective inattention, the process underlying all security operations, guarantees that we do not see—that we cannot say—whatever it is that would make us too anxious" (p. 108). That which can be neither seen nor talked about cannot be experienced. It is outside thought and feeling. It is, in other words, not known. In contrast to processes of repression, where known or knowable content is excluded from consciousness because awareness would generate unacceptable levels of conflict, selective inattention works much earlier in the processing sequence. The operating principle for selective inattention is that what is not noticed cannot be known, and if it is not known one does not have to deal with its emotional and personal consequences. For example, in infertility counseling, patients frequently selectively inattend those numbers having to do with the rates of success or failure for a procedure: "I never paid attention to statistics, I just figured the procedure would work for me."

Many times, such as when a couple ignores statistical information, it is easy to discern the presence of selective inattention and then to work with it. It is easy because the couple is selectively inattending and the clinician is not. We know the information—but not always. Often we too are in the dark. Sometimes, as illustrated in the lengthy case example of Susan and Chris, we are in the dark because the couple's selective inattention forecloses the exploration that would otherwise be needed to know what is going on. Other times we are in the dark for more personal reasons, such as when we ourselves are selectively inattending the clinically relevant information, and those selective inattentions organize our countertransferential experience. For example, while working with a young couple in their late-20s in which the wife had a diagnosis of POF (premature ovarian failure), I often found myself blithely unaware of her medical situation as they described yet one more alternative health reproductive option she had found on the web. These sessions would end and my head would snap back with the sudden recognition, completely absent during the session, that a particular herb or practice simply could not support all the hope we had been heaping on it.

I had selectively inattended the realistic probabilities of the interventions being discussed to avoid my own discomfort with this couple's situation; I really wanted to believe that everything would just work out for them. Selective inattention organized my response. But this was not a significant problem for the treatment. It would be so only if I tried to ignore my countertransference or act on it directly rather than trying to think with it. Thinking with it—asking myself, "What was I missing?" and using my countertransference as data and puzzle—helped me to explore with them the deep despair that needed to be crossed before they were able to consider donor gametes as an option.

In whatever form, selective inattention is a closed door, and you can never know what is behind it until you first recognize that you are, in fact, facing a closed door. It is neither an impenetrable wall nor a transparent pathway. Rather, the best way to see what is on the other side of the closed door is to open it. As already stated, countertransference reactions, both one's selective inattentions and one's responses to the couple's selective inattentions, can be useful indications that you are indeed facing a closed door with potentially useful information or activity on the other side.

Susan and Chris

In the following example, a man, Chris, was selectively inattending a basic, unspoken belief that if he just followed this or that dictate he would finally be able to earn the love and respect of his verbally abusive father. As he eventually said, "I had no idea part of wanting a kid was to get him finally to love me." Only after he began to formulate and discuss that belief was he able to move forward and energetically pursue the decision that he and his wife had made to adopt.

Susan and Chris were a happy couple. She was a successful, bohemian-type executive in advertising who was the adopted youngest of two older adopted siblings. He was the "golden boy," youngest of five of working-class parents. He, more through talent than hard work, had acquired an Ivy League MBA and was working successfully in the research/analytical end of investment banking. Before their marriage both of them knew that they were likely to have problems conceiving on their own because of medical problems Susan had experienced. They consulted with infertility specialists during the courtship and engagement, and this was when they were referred to me.

In this first phase of work together, it emerged that Chris's father was a verbally abusive, hard-drinking man who had tried to break up this otherwise happy and well-suited couple when he learned about the likelihood of infertility problems. His controlling cruelty included an especially ugly and hurtful episode in which he hired private investigators in an attempt to "dig up dirt" on Susan. The relationship between the couple and Chris's parents deteriorated to the point where Chris's parents were uninvited from the wedding when the father absolutely refused to apologize for his intrusion on Susan's privacy. Nevertheless, the wedding went forward and the marriage started happily, and several months after the honeymoon the treatment stopped.

Three years later, the couple returned. They had resumed some tentative contact with Chris's parents. There were occasional phone calls, and they no longer avoided going to the same family functions. However, there had not been any real rapprochement between them. At the time of this second contact, they had already spent 16 months in the "infertility bubble," which included several failed IVF cycles and one pregnancy that had raised their hopes but lasted only two months.

When they came back to treatment, Chris and Susan had had enough with technology, that is, Susan had. She was done and was ready to adopt. Being adopted herself and wanting now to be a mother, she was clear eyed and happy at the prospect of adoption. On the other hand, Chris had mixed feelings. He was clear that he wanted to raise a family and raise one with Susan, but he had questions about adoption. He just was not sure. So they actively sought out resources, went to conferences, attended an adoption support group, and explored their feelings in the couples treatment, especially their recognition of the importance to them of not having unequal genetic connections to their children. Donor gametes were not something they wanted. After a few months of work, he got to the point where he was ready. He felt all his questions and concerns had been addressed, and they decided to commit to adoption.

And that when the real trouble started. Susan wanted Chris to "carry the ball" on the adoption as she felt she had done during their time of unsuccessfully trying to get pregnant by using assisted reproductive technologies. Also, given his initial mixed feelings, she wanted to be sure he was not just "giving in." He very much wanted to give this to her. But the more they agreed on adoption, the more things he would forget to do, quite unlike his way of handling matters prior to the actual decision to adopt. Getting this or that paperwork done, calling a lawyer, arranging for a home visit, making a follow-up call to an agency were all things he said he would do—and then he wouldn't. Something would just interfere or he would forget. It was always something.

I thought there was still ambivalence to explore and, given our history of working well together, I assumed we would soon be able to work through the mixed feelings he was acting on rather than talking about. But this is not at all what happened; I could not have been more wrong. The sessions rapidly deteriorated into cycles of blame and shame, attack and defense. They would fight over the details of this or that undone task. She would accuse and he would defend. The harder she pushed, the more he apologized—and the less he did. They were stuck, and I was perplexed but still feeling pretty much within myself in the work we were doing.

Then they came in for a session in a good mood. She had reminded him several times during the week about contacting a lawyer and he had done it. While the situation was not optimal for them, since she felt she had to push him, they said they were now in a good place together, moving the process forward and not fighting as they had recently been doing.

As he started telling me about his good feelings about the work we had done to get to this point, feelings she said she shared, I found myself becoming increasingly annoyed with them. The more they talked and the more I listened, the more the annoyance began to turn to anger at his lack of initiative. I actually found myself wanting to find a phrase with which I could beat him over the head. I was thinking about slapping him around with accusations of fetishizing genetic information or of only pretending to care about Susan. Then I realized that, at least inside my head, which is where it belonged, I sort of sounded like his father—or at least like my image of his father. Caught in this countertransferential tumble, I wanted neither to act on it directly nor assume a one-to-one correspondence between the noise in my head and the clinical situation that needed attention. But the pull to do one of those two things was strong and incessant, like gravity. In order to find a way to work in the midst of this, I stood on the scaffolding of "What's not going on here?" and in that way extricated myself from the pull of the countertransferential experience, or at least I pulled myself far enough away to work. I really felt myself struggle to find a place to stand where I could try to engage Susan and Chris in an exploration of what was missing.

I said that the good feelings being expressed were interesting and an indication of their genuine caring and concern for each other; but I was wondering if perhaps they were working together not to learn what was troubling Chris, not to find out what was leading him not to take care of all the things he said he was going to do. I continued that perhaps there was an aspect of becoming a father this way, that is, through adoption, that Chris felt he could not explore because of fears that it might create too much anxiety either in him or in Susan, that the reality not being noticed would somehow make things feel unacceptably unsafe for the two of them.

Susan then commented with an angry laugh that it probably had something to do with that "bastard" (a name we all knew referred to his father). I said that, if it did, perhaps her anger at the father, however justified, might make it difficult for Chris to explore and discuss, even to notice, other kinds of feelings about his father and about becoming a father himself now that the two of them were on the edge of finally becoming parents. Susan said that even though she hated his father, she believed that Chris probably had other kinds of feelings as well. In response to a direct question from him, she said that, of course, she would not feel betrayed by those feelings; and if she did, it would be OK—she would know he really was not betraying her. As she said this, she turned to Chris and took his hand. With tears in his eyes, he said, "I don't know why, but I'm feeling really, really sad talking about this. I really don't like it." In what would happen frequently in the next few sessions, she reassured him that she loved him no matter how he felt about his father, "the bastard." Chris recognized that he had closed the door on noticing even the possibility of positive feelings about his father because of fears of betraying her and his own rage at the way his father had betrayed him.

Over the next few sessions, we were tentatively able to explore some of the good memories Chris had of time with his father and, more centrally, of his always feeling that his father responded not to him, but to his achievements, which came to him naturally and without much effort. In fact, what emerged was that *effort* was not approved; he received his father's effusive, and usually alcohol-inflected praise only for his easy "golden boy" achievements. But now, with adoption, effort was needed. He had to try, really, really try. And that was where he got stuck. Out of concern over betraying Susan, who had been so badly wounded by his father, and a previously unformulated identification with being the golden boy son his father wanted him to be, he had been selectively inattending to that aspect of his own desire to be a father that had to do with gaining his father's love and approval through easy, talent-based accomplishments. As he talked more about this, his desire for his father's love and approval, his sadness continued. In fact, it deepened for a time. Recognizing the lost possibility of winning his father's approval was a significant loss for him. He needed to mourn its loss. But at the same time his ability to take on the details of the adoption increased, as did his satisfaction in doing them.

Attention to my countertransferential annoyance and anger led me to ask, "What's not going on here?" and by asking that to begin a needed exploration of Chris's selective inattentions. Those difficult countertransferential moments suggested that together we were facing a closed door, and they were indeed difficult moments. It can be quite destabilizing to realize and think about seemingly nontherapeutic, even hostile, feelings about patients who have entrusted you with their care. Those feelings are, however, in a sense, inevitable and I believe our therapeutic responsibility is to think with them, not to ignore them or discharge them directly in action. It is by thinking with these uncomfortable inevitabilities that we can best help the couples who come to us for help.

SELECTIVE NONPARTICIPATION

Selective nonparticipation is a hybrid concept grown in the soil of ongoing efforts to make clinical use of countertransference experiences. It combines psychoanalytic and systemic approaches to understanding the clinical data generated while doing couples therapy. Brown (1993) stated: "The systemic approaches to couples and family therapy define problems as part of a repeating sequence of acts between several people (as opposed to conceiving of problems as a matter of meaning, or as a fit between expressions of each person's personality)." Selective nonparticipation draws from both these domains.

When working on the scaffolding of "What's not going on here?" it soon becomes apparent that selective inattention, as useful as it is, has limitations. Even stretching it as far as it can go does not mitigate the basic fact that its conceptual lineage as a psychoanalytic concept, even one from interpersonal psychoanalysis, which takes the most fully contextualized view possible of the individual mind, keeps it from providing all the conceptual help an engaged couples therapist needs. Selective inattention is limited to the individual-in-relation and the various psychological processes, such as attention and the construction of meaning, that help us create sufficiently safe and satisfying feelings of connectedness.

But in couples work much more is not going on. Selective inattention does not adequately address all those instances when the couple-as-a-system, or the couple-as-a-microculture, depending on one's preferred metaphor, was missing this or that interactional format or frame or relational ritual. Here, the omission of clinical interest is at the level of participation or action, not attention. Clinical relevance is in what the people were doing, or not doing, rather than what they were experiencing or not experiencing. Selective nonparticipation is a concept minted in attempts to get at this system-level reality in which couples manage their shared anxiety and collective security by not doing this or that to or with each other. In other words, they achieve sufficiently safe and satisfying feelings of connectedness; that is, they remain ensconced in the system, in their own marital microculture, by selectively not participating in some format, frame, or ritual. Unfortunately, what they are not doing is often what causes all the trouble.

Let me illustrate with an example, albeit one in which the selective nonparticipation registered first not as a countertransferential shadow but instead was discerned through inquiry and observation. In the following example of selective nonparticipation, the couple did not participate in a particular interactional format because, for them, to do so would have been to act outside the mutually constructed and accepted boundaries of their marriage and would have left them feeling unacceptably unsafe and abandoned.

They were successful artists with a loving and passionate, at times turbulent, relationship. Their fights would escalate as first one would flash and then the other. Soon there was screaming and rapid and verbally vicious escalations. Both ended up saying things they later regretted. Several years previously they had been in couples therapy for eight to ten sessions for work they described as primarily focused on communications skills. They were seeking additional help at the suggestion of the reproductive center where they would soon have their first IVF cycle. The way they framed it when they started with me was that they wanted help with their fighting. They both knew they should just walk away; they had learned that in the communications skills therapy, but they never did walk away and the fights continued. They understood the stresses of IVF and the hoped-for strains that would accompany becoming parents and wanted, finally, to get a handle on their arguments.

I was intrigued by the fact that, even though they both "knew better," they seemed to be selectively nonparticipating in what could be called a "cool-down" format or frame. They really knew that nothing was resolved by fighting, that exploring and arguing were mutually exclusive. They also knew that one or both should just go to a different room to cool off rather than stand toe-to-toe and exchange verbal blows. But they always stood and fought.

What emerged from several weeks of exploration was that escalation, within the specific microculture of this marriage, was a powerful bond and cooling-off was experienced as an abandonment. We explored this pattern through many different domains and specific examples. In their creative work, lovemaking, cooking, charity involvements, and even family-of-origin connections, each always tried to outdo the other. Upping the ante and games of emotional chicken—who would bail out first (and, of course, neither would)—was their way. And for them, it mostly worked. Their relationship was built on these escalating, feedback-looping affect-state transformations, but only in one direction: more stimulation, more excitement. It was always about more, about taking the initial condition and pushing it as far as they could make it go.

They began to see that they never participated in the other direction together. Even their preferred modes of relaxation, he with classical music and she with their dog, were separate from each other. They never did "less" together. Always more. And, in fighting, where they knew one of them should try and cool things down, their pattern of escalation was causing problems. They eventually concluded that if one were to try and cool down a fight, it would feel like a violation of their basic marital agreement. It would be for them an unacceptable abandonment.

With this understanding in hand, and often given explicit voice by one or the other as a fight escalated, they were able to start participating in the previously absent "cool-down" format. Rather than flashing with anger, one of them would reassure the other that he or she was not abandoning the other but was just choosing not to fight. Cooling down even became an opportunity for escalation as they would humorously compete to see who was more of the peacemaker. Participating in the previously absent cooldown format significantly reduced the frequency of their destructive arguments and helped them begin to solve many of the solvable problems that previously would be lost in the static of ongoing argumentation.

That example is a useful illustration of the concept of selective nonparticipation. Let us now explore some of its complexities. Let me note that working on the scaffolding of "what's not going here?" obviously requires that we keep in mind some notion of what is possible, of what a couple could be seeing or doing if they were not defensively inattending and nonparticipating. But there are both a danger and a challenge in this obvious requirement to delimit the possible.

A clinical approach that uses the possible as a scaffolding for thinking with countertransference experiences can easily, and unhelpfully, be confused with telling people what they should be doing or seeing. This is, I think, a danger. A walk through any chain bookstore, or a click through the online version, rapidly reveals an overabundance of experts, all selling books and tapes telling people what they should do or how they should live their lives. In sharp but subtle contrast, paying attention to the presence of selective inattention and selective nonparticipation is not about imposing one's standards for experience and action. It is about trying to help each couple expand their range of what is knowable and doable. Of course, one must recognize that, for a couple straddling technocultural fault lines, what is knowable and doable may be outside or different from one's own repertoire. In other words, it is about their *could*, not our *should*; about possibility and not normativity.

But what does it look like in clinical terms to say that as therapists we need to keep our curiosity focused on what is possible for the specific couple with whom one is working rather than on what may be normative from our own frame of reference? A frequently encountered and clear illustration of focusing on possibility and not normativity comes from working with couples with deeply held religious beliefs different from one's own.

For example, I worked with a recently married Orthodox Jewish couple, modern enough to see a secular therapist but still deeply observant. He was infertile following treatment for testicular cancer just prior to the wedding. They came with questions: Should they divorce? Should they adopt? What for me was a simple technical solution, donor insemination, was for them an impossibility. They had had several consultations with trusted rabbis and were clear that donor sperm violated their religious beliefs and was not even on the table for discussion. I am trying here to highlight that this couple cannot be seen to be selectively nonparticipating in a discussion of donor sperm or selectively inattending to its possibilities, any more than someone not seeing infrared radiation is selectively inattending to something outside the possibilities of our visual system. Donor sperm was not in the realm of possibility for this couple. Thus, when I found myself frightened for the future of these two gentle, caring persons who had already developed a deep bond for each other and asked myself, "What's not going on here?" I tried to make sure my thinking went in the direction of this couple's possibilities, and not my own.

What was missing, as subsequent work showed, was any discussion of the wife's deep sadness and loss over pregnancy and her anger over the fact that his medical problems had deprived her of opportunities for childbirth. These feelings were never discussed because of her fear of hurting him, her fear of not being a kind and supportive wife. But she knew that she felt them. And he knew it too, which also became apparent once they began to participate in a discussion of both their shared and their individual grief. Prior to their therapeutic work there had been no discussion of these shared affect-states; both were selectively nonparticipating in any verbalized recognition that they each felt loss and anger. I should note that after mourning the loss of biological children, he offered her the option of a divorce. She declined, and instead they energetically began to pursue adoption.

That example illustrates how imposing one's normative standards for behavior can become a danger when one is working on the scaffolding of "What's not going on here?" But the central challenge remains: how do we know what is possible? What is the range of formats, frames, and rituals in which couples can participate? How do we see or hear or otherwise relate to that which is not present? In what might a couple be selectively nonparticipating? Clearly, one's own history of interpersonal relations, clinical experience, empathic capacity, and willingness to tolerate the anxiety and uncertainty of decentering from personally familiar interactions plays a significant role when one is trying to engage the absent but still possible.

In addition, especially when one is using countertransferences as experiences to think with, ongoing supervision can significantly deepen one's engagement with the possible. But I also find it useful to "hit the books." For the more empirically minded, this might become a search for an elusive comprehensive typology of marital interactions. For those with a more literary sensibility, questions concerning the range of the possible would be answered by having a rich repertoire of stories and a supple imagination to process them. While the former would look to Erving Goffman for guidance, the latter might turn to John Irving or some other novelist, poet, or playwright whose work illuminates what people can do to and with each other. My own thinking is that both offer important ways of knowing about the possible and each is useful to expand the range of possible marital and relational interactions to which one has access.

Being a committed pragmatist, I try to use whatever I can when formulating possible answers for the question, "In what interactions might this couple be selectively nonparticipating?" Everything can help. In the following example, I used observational research findings as a way to work on the scaffolding of "What's not going on here?" John Gottman (1979, 1980, 1993, 1999) and his research associates (Gottman and Krokoff, 1989; Gottman and Levenson, 1999; Gottman and Silver, 1999) have been doing quasi-naturalistic couples observational research for many years. One method they use is bringing couples into their "lab" to live for a weekend so the research team can record and then study their interactions. The researchers do this over a period of years and then correlate specific interactions with other variables. Doing so allows them to discern interactive routines that can be correlated with such measures as marital satisfaction, as well as those kinds of interactions that lead eventually to despair or divorce.

Although many questions remain about the psychometric properties, theoretical foundations, and clinical applicability of observational couples research (for a review, see Heyman, 2001), I have found that this developing research tradition delineates the functional consequences of different interactive routines in a way that significantly enriches the range of missing possibilities I have in mind when I ask, "What's not going on here?" For example, Gottman and his associates (Gottman and Krokoff, 1989; Gottman and Levenson, 1999; Gottman and Silver, 1999) have found that the reliable appearance of rituals of repair following conflict are better predictors of marital satisfaction than is either the frequency or the severity of the conflict. In other words, though making-up may be hard to do, it is also an indication of a healthy marriage, as illustrated by my example of the two artists committed to each other and to escalation.

Another set of interactions highly correlated with martial satisfaction can be called friendship rituals. These include, among others, a deepening knowledge of the details of each other's daily life, nurturing camaraderie in pursuit of shared goals, and developing empathy rather than contempt for the other when differences are encountered. While marriage is more than being friends, marital satisfaction does seem to require a solid friendship.

Kathy and Paul

The following clinical vignette describes my responding to an uncomfortable countertransferential experience of lifelessness in the midst of drama by thinking with the possibilities described by Gottman, specifically this couple's selective nonparticipation in those friendship rituals. This couple, among other things, selectively nonparticipated in conversations about the experiences of their day because doing so brought their children's significant medical and developmental problems so sharply into focus that neither could bear it. They were in a sense protecting themselves and each other by fighting rather than talking. The therapy helped them to understand and then slowly to undermine the implicit agreement they made that it is better to become distant and estranged than it would be to confront unfathomably deep feelings of loss, disappointment, and rage.

Kathy and Paul, two ambitious, driven, highly successful persons from extraordinarily accomplished, complicated family backgrounds, met when they were in their mid-30s and decided to marry. Both before and after marriage they lived the "good life" and after a few years decided to have a child. Infertility was their first shock, and a big shock it was. Their adult identity included great pride in the fact that through talent and hard work they had achieved significant success in pretty much everything they had ever done as adults. Infertility really shook them. In the midst of a second IVF cycle they had their second shock: triplets. Finally, there was a third shock, significant medical and developmental problems in all three children. Their son died at two months, and they were referred to me when their daughters were 20 months.

They presented a picture, consistent with their histories, of having everything about their daughters' care perfectly organized with the best of everything: the best treatments, the best help, the best technology. Except life was now painfully problematic. It was "hell." They were fighting all the time. Bad fights. He would complain and criticize until she exploded. Or Kathy would shut down emotionally, becoming hypercompetent and organized until Paul exploded. Their sex life had evaporated. Things were deteriorating, and, by the time we started, it was their shared stubbornness, more than anything else, that held them together. And they were not at all sure they even wanted to stay together. But they did agree that if they divorced they wanted to split in the best way possible for their daughters.

Each had been through previous individual therapy and was quite fluent discussing the emotional dynamics of their relationship, such as Paul's perceptions of Kathy's similarities to his mother and Kathy's perceptions of Paul's similarities to her father. She had always feared she would end up with another work-obsessed man who preferred career to family life and he wanted a woman whose emotional availability was constant and not tied to complicated relationship contingencies.

When therapy began, Kathy claimed that she now "knew" him to be the man she feared, and Paul no longer felt that she could be the woman he wanted. But these historical explorations did not gather any momentum, and I was soon witness (referee?) to their often contemptuous arguments. After one session in which Paul defensively said that he probably never loved Kathy at all, she came in to the next session armed with a stack of love letters and demanded to know if he was a liar then or now. Clearly, this was nasty revisionist history, a microculture war at its hurtful worst. Although I knew this was a marriage in trouble, the contempt in the room was thick enough to cut with a knife; my internal response to this dramatic confrontation was a surprising and uncomfortable feeling of lifelessness, a deadness strikingly at odds with the drama of the moment. As I listened to the ensuing point–counterpoint attack-and-parry and to the discordant notes of my own lifeless listening, I began to think that perhaps the lifelessness of my listening was a clue to their selective nonparticipation in some other kind of interaction.

So, standing again on the platform of "What's not going on here?" I decided to interrupt their attempt at revising the entire history of their relationship to make it consistent with their current awful feelings. I commented that they had shared their fights with me and that I had witnessed their ability to hurt each other, despite my efforts to contain them. Also, I had witnessed discussions of objective, practical matters having to do with their daughters' various treatments.

I went on that I wondered if those interactions, taken together accurately defined the boundaries of their entire relationship. Was it really now all a matter of practical arrangements, fights, and hurting each other? And had it always been that way? When they asked me what I meant, with Gottman's work firmly in mind, I commented that, among all the other things now missing from their marriage, it seemed they no longer just talked as friends. They then recalled that they used to come together for cocktails and go over the details of each other's day. They would describe what they did, whom they talked to, the problems they encountered, and how they either solved them or didn't. But since the infertility and the birth of their children, they did things like that less and less frequently. And they stopped altogether when their son died. When they asked me if it was important that they start communicating again as they had, I said it probably was but that what was most important was to understand why they stopped doing something they both enjoyed and that worked so well for them. I went on that it may have just been that there was no time, but it was also possible that they stopped being friends for important emotional reasons that needed to be understood.

In the weeks and months that followed, we explored what it would mean for them to go back to engaging each other as friends. We discovered that it would mean regaining openness and respect for the subjectivity of the other, including having to confront all they had lost, something neither felt was possible. It became apparent that they were indeed selectively nonparticipating for very good reasons. Not only had they lost their son and lost the "good life" they loved, one that was supposed to include play dates, child-focused fashion and travel, private schools, and all the rest, they both also felt they had lost part of their identity. Accepting their spouse as a friend now meant accepting that they both had in his or her own way, failed as people. And they could not make such an admission.

As the treatment slowly progressed, they worked through the recognition that reengaging was terrifying because they were trying to protect themselves—and each, to a degree, the other—from the harsh realities of their current situation. Working-through was by no means a smooth or linear process. It included a trial separation that led to a decision to work things out because "being apart was even worse." It has been several years since Kathy and Paul came to my office, and they continue to try to grow closer, to find ways to use the other as a source of comfort and pleasure, albeit now with a bond knit from loss and grief, rather than being bound together mainly by the pleasures of the "good life."

In that example, as Gottman's research suggests, "something" was not going on that I could think with when I was caught in my uncomfortable countertransferential moment of lifelessness in the midst of drama. Attending to these selective nonparticipations helped us move the process forward so that they could further process their significant grief and personal loss and go on to try and resurrect their marriage. I want to point out, though, that empirical observations of marital interactions are just one of several research traditions I find useful when working on the scaffolding of "What's not going here?" Developmental research, specifically microanalysis of parent–infant interactions pioneered by, among others, Stern (1985), Kaye (1982), Beebe and Lachmann (2002), and Bruner (1983), has proved extremely useful in describing affectively rich interactional formats, the absence of which may be significant for understanding what is not going on with a couple. In fact, any approach that studies mutually coconstructed systems of experience and action can be useful additions to the scaffolding of "What's not going on here?"

CAVEATS AND CONCLUSIONS

I have presented countertransference as intrinsically neither virtue nor vice but as an inevitability that can be useful when treated as an experience to think with, its value depending on what we do with it. In an effort to make it easier for you to think with countertransference, I described the conceptual framework I use, the scaffolding of "What's not going on here?" It provides a conceptual place to stand so one can more easily consider processes of selective inattention and selective nonparticipation. I have further suggested and tried to illustrate that those processes often register first in countertransference experiences.

However, the hindsight of clinical writing is 20/20 and may obscure some of the original difficulty. By its very nature, countertransference is difficult to think with, and this difficulty may have been obscured in the service of providing clear examples. Countertransference can indeed be compelling and difficult to recognize. In fact, it becomes more compelling, more insistent the more it is not recognized. It is, in many ways, like Verbal Kint's warning about Keyser Soze in *The Usual Suspects*, a movie as clinically fascinating as it is entertaining (Essig and DiNardo, 1996): "The greatest trick the devil ever played on humanity was convincing us he doesn't exist." Countertransference can be such a trickster. When it convinces us it does not exist, it can indeed become devilish. Useful when thought with, devilish when ignored. So, for both caveat and in conclusion, let me say that the only countertransference to worry about is the one you think does not exist. If in the course of your work with couples dealing with infertility you ever feel yourself free from difficult countertransferential experiences, then that is precisely the time to seek out supervision!

Throughout this chapter I have focused on specific moments when thinking with countertransference allowed access to previously unformulated inattentions and nonparticipations. But I do not want to leave you with the impression that those moments were keystones in seamless arches of change. The moments discussed, though illustrating processes of selective inattention and selective nonparticipation, often registering first in my countertransference, were only some of many moments when those processes were noted and discussed, sometimes clued by countertransference and other times not. If your work feels messier than my examples, please know that mine does too.

I want to close by making explicit my assumptions about personal experience and shared interactions—in other words, the individual and the system. The overall systemic organization of what couples do to and with each other has functional consequence for the organization of each person's experience. At the same time, changes in feeling-state, self-organization, and personal experience of either person in a marriage has functional consequences for the overall system. The functional organization of each includes the other. Each constructs, not only influences, the other, as well as operating by principles unique to its own domain. There is a constant oscillation between the individual-in-the-marriage and the marriage-in-the-individual. By listening for both selective inattention and selective nonparticipation, we increase the chances of finding what needs to be found so that we can better help couples move from the often painful simplicities of darkness and imprisonment to the complexities and challenges of knowledge and freedom.

REFERENCES

Beebe, B. & Lachmann, F. M. (2002), *Infant Research and Adult Treatment: Co-constructing Interactions.* Hillsdale, NJ: The Analytic Press.

Bromberg, P. (1998), *Standing in the Spaces: Essays on Clinical Process, Trauma, and Dissociation.* Hillsdale, NJ: The Analytic Press.

Brown, L. (1993), The interpersonal analyst as couples therapist: Finding one's way with double vision. Presented at panel on "The Interpersonal Analyst and the Couple: How Does it Work?" William Alanson White Society Special Interest Group Meeting, New York City, May.

Bruner, J. S. (1983), *Child's Talk: Learning to Use Language.* New York: Norton.

Burns, L. H. & Covington, S. N. (1999), *Infertility Counseling; A Comprehensive Handbook for Clinicians.* New York: Parthenon.

Essig, T. S. & DiNardo, A. C. (1996), Truth is more than verbal. Presented at meeting of NYU Psychoanalysis and Humanities Group, New York City, Nov. 14.

Gottman, J. M. (1979), *Marital Interaction: Experimental Investigations.* New York: Academic Press.

——— (1980), Consistency of nonverbal affect and affect reciprocity in marital interaction. *J. Consult. Clin. Psychol.*, 48:711–717.

——— (1993), The roles of conflict engagement, escalation, and avoidance in marital interaction: A longitudinal view of five types of couples. *J. Consult. Clin. Psychol.*, 61:6–15.

——— (1999), *The Marriage Clinic: A Scientifically Based Marital Therapy.* New York: Norton.

——— & Krokoff, L. J. (1989), Marital interaction and satisfaction: A longitudinal view. *J. Consult. Clin. Psychol.*, 57:47–52.

——— & Levenson, R. W. (1999), How stable is marital interaction over time? *Family Process*, 38:143–158.

——— & Silver, N. (1999), *The Seven Principles for Making Marriage Work.* New York: Three Rivers Press.

Heyman, R. E. (2001), Observation of couple conflicts: Clinical assessment applications, stubborn truths, and shaky foundations. *Psycholog. Assess.*, 13:5–35.

Kaye, K. (1982), *The Mental and Social Life of Babies: How Parents Create Persons.* Chicago: University of Chicago Press.

Lionells, M. Fiscalini, J. Mann, C. & Stern, D. B. (1995), *Handbook of Interpersonal Psychoanalysis*, Hillsdale, NJ: The Analytic Press.

Meyers, M., Diamond, R., Kezur, D., Scharf, C., Weinshel, M. &, Rait, D. S. (1995), An infertility primer for family therapists. *Family Process*, 34:219–229.

―――― Weinshel, M., Scharf, C., Kezur, D., Diamond, R. & Rait, D. S. (1995), An infertility primer for family therapists, II: Working with couples who struggle with infertility. *Family Process*, 34:231–240.

Papp, P., ed. (2002), *Couples on the Fault Line: New Directions for Therapists*. New York: Guilford Press.

Rosen, A. (2003), Honing my thoughts about cloning. Mental Health Professional Interest Group Newsletter. American Society of Reproductive Medicine, Fall Issue.

Stammer, H., Wischmann, T. & Verres, R. (2002), Counseling and couple therapy for infertile couples. *Family Process*, 41:111–122.

Stern, D. B. (1995), Cognition and language. In: *Handbook of Interpersonal Psychoanalysis*, ed. J. Fiscalini, C. H. Mann & D. B. Stern. Hillsdale, NJ: The Analytic Press.

Stern, D. N. (1985), *The Interpersonal World of the Infant: A View from Psychoanalysis and Developmental Psychology*. New York: Basic Books.

7

FROM INFERTILITY TO ADOPTION

Anne F. Malavé

*I*n order to work within the overlapping space of infertility and adoption, therapists must be willing to participate in powerful and disturbing vortexes of emotion, as their patients grapple with profound, primitive, and existential dilemmas and make crucial life choices.

MY CLINICAL APPROACH

I wish to acknowledge explicitly some of my beliefs. I believe that people are individuals and that they will inevitably experience both infertility and adoption in similar as well as in powerfully unique and different ways. I believe that the therapist's values are *always* a present and powerful influence, and I try to be as aware as possible of my own values. I also understand that a full awareness of unconscious dynamics is never possible and that what we can talk about, or become aware of, is always incomplete.

When I begin to work with people, I clarify with them how I see my role in helping them, including what I do and what I do not do. I also tell them something about the way I work, which I find to be helpful and reassuring. I tell people that I see my role as one of helping them to explore how their infertility has affected and is affecting them, of helping them to understand themselves, and of helping them to find their own path forward, either toward more medical treatments, adoption, parenting through third-party reproduction, or remaining child free. I tell them that by exploring adoption, I aim to help them understand the psychological issues and the important *differences*, as well as the *similarities*, of this family-building option.

I clarify that I do *not* see my role as being the sole source of their education about adoption, although some of what we do together will be educational. I advise them to do reading and research on adoption and to seek out and talk to adoptive parents. I also clarify that I do not see my role as one of helping them to adopt, or to teach them what I call "the how to's," or "the nuts and bolts" of the adoption process. Toward this end, I advise them to research adoption carefully and to take advantage of the many excellent books on the subject (see Johnston, 1992; Melina, 1998). I may warn them that there are unscrupulous and exploitative people in the field of adoption, and at times I directly advise them to slow down and get more information about one approach or another.

I always recommend that people join adoption support groups such as The Adoptive Parents Committee and attend their meetings. I sometimes recommend lawyers and other adoption professionals, and I suggest that they attend conferences, workshops, and seminars. And I refer people to Resolve, The National Infertility Association.

DISCLOSURE

I share very little personal information about myself with the people I work with, and I do not disclose my personal experiences in the areas of infertility, adoption, reproduction, and parenting. When asked, I explain that the reason for this approach is that the treatment is for them to discover what is right for *them*, not *me*. I point out to them that they have probably already felt great pressure from many different sources, including medical professionals, family, friends, other people experiencing infertility, and the larger society, and that I aim to provide them with a *safe* space that is as free as possible from outside pressures for them to discover what is right for them, which I do not believe is possible if they know the personal choices that I have made. Generally, my impression is that people feel reassured by this approach, and sometimes they explicitly tell me that they asked me *because* they feared that I would "have an agenda" and would influence them in one direction or another. Naturally, there are other people who are looking for someone to tell them what to do and who may be disappointed or even angry at this stance.

I do disclose some of the thoughts and feelings that I have during sessions. In my work, I depend heavily on visual imagery, which is partly reflective of the way my mind works and also as the result of these "visual metaphors" enhancing my clinical work by providing an immediacy and affective resonance and power ("a picture is worth a thousand words"). Usually these images are individual and arise spontaneously during my work as the result of my experience of a particular interaction with a person or couple. Sometimes I have "general metaphors" that I use again and again. The "bridge" between infertility and adoption is one of them.

I find the metaphor of the *bridge* very useful when I am helping people who are considering adoption. Implicit in this image are many different meanings and possibilities. For one thing, I believe that this bridge metaphor allows people the freedom to take the first steps to what is usually an overwhelming and difficult endeavor without feeling that they have to commit themselves to this option. This makes the exploration of adoption, often described as "another roller-coaster ride, just like infertility," both possible and manageable. Some people may start this journey, but they do not "cross over" to become adoptive parents. Crossing over is not a requirement, and people can move to and fro freely, venturing forward, and then retreating, at their own pace. I usually frame any beginning discussion of adoption as an "exploration" of the similarities and differences in parenting through adoption, and I use the bridge metaphor as a way of capturing the idea of the transition to a new and different path of family building.

The journey across the bridge is made in the same way that all psychological change occurs and is negotiated in a series of steps forward and backward, in shifts to and fro, retracing one's steps and then regaining momentum, as working through leads to new ground. There is no prescribed timeline, and, in fact, each journey is unique. For each person choosing this path, there is a developmental process involved, and I believe that, regardless of whether or not the bridge is crossed, this exploration will help people move forward in their own personal journey through infertility. I believe that therapists can be the guides and provide the necessary "holding space" (Winnicott, 1971) within which this journey can be successfully navigated.

AT THE BEGINNING OF THE BRIDGE

Before someone actively decides to explore adoption, the *idea* of adoption has long been present, in one way or another, since infertility began. For I believe that there is no one who is experiencing infertility who has *not*, at one time or other, at least *thought* about adoption as an option. Adoption is ever-present in the experience of infertility, even if only as a rejected path, or as a club that the individual or couple has no interest in joining. By the time people are talking about it as an option, there has already been an important shift. But even if they are not talking about it, the idea of adoption is constantly offered from the outside by well-meaning others. "You can always adopt" is a refrain so familiar to people experiencing infertility that it frequently seems to follow them like an unwelcome shadow that they cannot shake. They hear it from all who know about their infertility, from well-meaning loved ones, coworkers, and neighbors, each of whom may suggest this option as though it were an easy solution that has not yet been considered by the person or couple experiencing the infertility. It is frequently presented upon hearing the news of the infertility and is almost always offered when the people experiencing infertility are at their lowest, such as after a failed IVF cycle.

"You can always adopt" can seem insensitive and painful and is experienced by some as an *assault*. It can be experienced as (or may be intended to mean), "You do not have the right to continue treatment" or "People like you have to settle for second best." People struggling with infertility often come to dread those words and the inexplicably intense feelings of pain and anger that these words arouse in them. In fact, often this kind of quick response is the very reason that many people are reluctant to disclose their infertility. For, although adoption can represent *hope* for some people struggling with infertility, before that can happen it is more likely to be experienced as something to be *dreaded*, as a *threat*, associated with the one thing that they fear the most: acknowledgment that treatment has failed and banishment from the world that they have known and longed for (i.e., the world where people are biologically related to their children).

"Why don't you adopt? Then you'll get pregnant!" is another common refrain. Despite the research on conception after adoption, which indicates that there is no greater probability of becoming pregnant after adoption than before, much of the general public is misinformed about this possibility, as well as about adoption in general. They believe it to be, for example, quick, inexpensive, and simple—all of which are not true. This comment implies that the goal is to have a biological child and that adoption is a "consolation prize," which may very much be the way that people approaching adoption feel at the beginning of their journey.

When people arrive at the point where they start to explore adoption, they are often physically and emotionally drained and demoralized, and this whole area may be associated with inadequacy and compromise. At this point, turning to adoption may become synonymous with "giving up," "defeat," and "personal failure."

Typically, people do a fair amount of soul searching as they consider exploring this route. Here are some of the comments I often hear: "Why would I want a stranger in my home?" "All adopted kids are messed up, and people who adopt are all weird." "Everyone else in the clinic was going to continue, no matter what it might take. . . . I felt like I was betraying them."

In short, the beginning of the bridge is dominated by the experience of infertility. People bring with them to adoption the legacy of their infertility: the shame, anxiety, depression, diminished self-esteem, isolation, loneliness, and the loss of control. They may have a *tunnel vision*, where the result of seeing outcomes in terms of success or failure has narrowed their focus to seeing a biological child, the fantasized "perfect child," as their only chance at success. The loss of this biological child, this long-desired for perfection, is sometimes experienced by people who cannot conceive as "dooming" them to failure. These feelings of failure are often projected onto adoption, which is often seen as the "poor cousin" of infertility options. In my experience, these experiences of the "lost perfect child" and the feelings of failure and the distaste and rejection of imperfection follow some people who have experienced infertility as they move into the world of adoption. This legacy of infertility may be manifest in various ways, from projecting feelings of personal failure onto the adopted child and the birth mother, to having feelings of entitlement to compensation for the losses and difficulties they have sustained during the infertility, to a desire for perfection in a different form—the perfect adoption.

People who are at the beginning of their adoption exploration are usually concerned with the possibility of adopting a child as close as possible to the child that they would have had biologically. They are interested in the *similarities* between having a child biologically and through adoption, and many want to minimize or deny differences. This is a time when one hears statements like: "My cousin was adopted, and she isn't different." "My friends (or relatives, or neighbors, or colleagues) have adopted, and their child is just like them; you'd never know he or she was adopted."

Although these statements may be understood as a denial of the differences of adoption, I think they are also attempts to *connect*, to make adoption personal, to integrate the idea of adoption, which is often a *foreign* idea, with something familiar. I use these statements as opportunities to explore adoption, and I often frame this exploration as looking at "similarities *and* differences." In fact, I believe that an important part of adoption exploration has to do with exploring all previous experiences with adoption.

Other attempts to integrate adoption may be more difficult for professionals to hear, such as when the child is seen as a *commodity*. Here are some frequent comments that I find more difficult: "I love my cats, so I guess I could love an adopted child." "I'd just love to adopt one of those little Chinese babies. They're so cute!" "I feel disgusted by the idea of adoption. Who would want someone else's garbage?"

Many people pursue adoption and infertility treatments simultaneously, which means that the decision to adopt is separate from the decision to end medical treatment. In some cases, pursuing both paths at the same time makes it more difficult for people to understand the importance of grieving the infertility, a process that may be delayed until after the adoption has been completed. When people are moving along both pathways simultaneously, I encourage them to choose between the two when the possibility of a placement is close, so that they can have sufficient time with the adopted child before another child possibly enters the family. Other people want reassurance that they can adopt and then return for more treatments, which may or may not be related to a lack of acceptance of the adoption. I encourage people to consider how returning for treatment might affect their adopted child. I explain that returning to infertility treatment *immediately* after adoption raises some concern that they have not given themselves enough time to get to know their child and to adjust to parenting. I also try to get people to consider spacing between siblings and the possible meanings to the adopted child that their parents continued to pursue having a biological child shortly after adopting them.

At the beginning, many people want to move straight ahead toward adoption without stopping, so that they can avoid feeling the loss of the biological child and to ignore or deny the realities of adoption, which they find hard to face, particularly the existence of the birth parents. It is important to help people grieve. I have generally found that helping is easier with couples, where usually one member is more in touch with and more eager to explore the loss than the other. I find that people have great difficulty considering the reality of the birth parents; most people are terrified by the idea of any contact with them and see their existence as a *threat*. The birth mother is often experienced as particularly threatening, especially by the infertile woman, who often feels intense feelings of competition with the (fertile) birth mother.

It is very difficult for people experiencing infertility and who have struggled so hard to have a biological child to imagine the difficulty birth parents face and how they could "give up" their biological child. It is not uncommon for prospective adoptive parents to disparage birth parents. I try to help people with their many fears of rejection, replacement, and competition and to help prospective adoptive parents understand that how they feel toward the birth parents will have an important impact on their adopted child. I find that it is extremely hard for prospective adoptive parents to imagine what achieving an integrated understanding of adoption would be like when it is all so new and when the differences loom so large.

From the beginning, adoption is experienced as a private and personal, as well as a public and social, event concerning significant others, such as partners, family, and friends, and also the public at large. People considering adoption have the reactions of other people strongly in mind and, from the beginning, consider what this might mean, in terms of issues of disclosure, privacy, and being different. I find that people who are beginning to explore adoption have great anxiety about the home-study process and even more anxiety about sharing information with birth parents. I see that fears about open adoption often drive decision making, and in my experience it is rare at this point for people to be open to either open adoption or the idea of openness in adoption. People who have experienced infertility are no strangers to struggles with disclosure, but they need help to understand how adoption information also belongs to the adopted child. It is very important to help prospective adoptive parents imagine the consequences of how they treat information (both by disclosing and also in terms of the importance of *acquiring* information) for an adopted child.

Approaches to adoption are as varied as the people themselves: some people carefully investigate multiple pathways, while others wait to turn to adoption until they get some definitive ending, they use up all their money, or they burn out, emotionally and psychologically, from infertility treatments. Many prefer not to slow down to learn about adoption; they move as quickly as they can to get to their goal of having a child. These people are not likely to present themselves for treatment, but, if they are already in existing treatments, their therapists can try to encourage them to slow down, to familiarize themselves with this new territory.

The decision to pursue adoption is often driven by one member of a couple (usually, but not always, the woman), while the other is undecided, unclear, more ambivalent, or even downright against the idea. Rarely do couples make the same decisions or feel the same emotions about infertility and adoption at the same time, and it can be enormously reassuring to point out this discrepancy, as well as to imply that, for most couples, agreement can be successfully negotiated.

In couples work, it can be enormously helpful to stress the importance of agreement, as well as to help couples understand how they work as a "system," each holding a piece of their combined experience and often balancing the other—for example, one person holding the hope, while the other takes a more skeptical approach. I have found it to be crucial in working with couples where one partner is reluctantly being "dragged along" to insist that we have a period of exploration, a "space" or "time out" from taking action, so they can familiarize themselves with the emotional issues of adoption. I point out the contribution of each person, and sometimes I find myself saying things like, "Well, a car needs an accelerator as well as a brake to function." This intervention is often an important part of my establishing a working relationship with the "reluctant" partner, who is most likely to see me as an ally of the partner who is moving ahead more rapidly toward adoption. Often the more reluctant partner is the man, who may expect me to ally with another woman more easily than with him. It can be very helpful to remind couples how they came to agreement about previous decisions during infertility treatment or earlier in their marriages. It is also important to point out how far they have come until this point and to remind them that it has been a *process*, and that more changes may be expected along the way.

Although the idea of adoption is difficult and intimidating, most people view it as leading to a child with more certainty than infertility treatments do and also as a way of taking back control (there is much that people can do to make an adoption happen, and happen faster). Turning to adoption can rekindle *hope*, of becoming parents, but also of finding a way to move forward from what has been, for many people, a period of painful *stuckness* in their lives. With this hope, and this move forward, can come a very great relief and a move toward a redefinition of identity and life purpose. As in any crisis, there is always great opportunity for change and personal growth. I have found that these more positive feelings are often dependent on whether or not the decisions to adopt and to end treatment have been made: for some people, these decisions are linked, whereas for others they are separate. The decision to adopt is usually accompanied by hope, and the decision to end medical treatment is often accompanied by an enormous sense of relief.

It is well known that people experience infertility according to their own personality styles (Goldfarb, Rosenthal, and Utian,

1985). For example, the person who is obsessive experiences infertility as a punishment for letting things get out of control, and the avoidant person sees it as a dangerous invasion of privacy. In my experience, these same personality styles powerfully affect the relationship between the patient and the therapist. The obsessive patient experiences the therapist as *critical*, and the avoidant person sees the therapist as *intrusive*.

The path to adoption is filled with sadness and loss as well as with redefinition and great gain. While working in this area, I find myself feeling at the extremes, from great satisfaction and joy, to great despair, sadness, and helplessness. While most recognize the *hallmark* of infertility as that of "loss of control," I find it useful to consider the powerful presence of "stuckness." I consider it a privilege to "make a difference" by helping people who have felt trapped inwardly by painful feelings, and outwardly by painful medical procedures, to move out of isolation, to take back control, and to *move forward*, whether toward adoption or in some other direction.

THE RACE TO ADOPTION

Many prefer not to slow down to learn about adoption; they are in too much pain, they are too *desperate*, they fear that they will not be able to move forward if they stop to take a look at the issues they will face. Many keep moving to avoid such feelings as grief and loss. As in medical treatments when people find it less painful to focus on procedures and statistics, so do people approaching adoption often focus on the "how to's" instead of on the feelings. Sometimes people enter headlong into this territory at the fastest speed, seeing only the "child at the end of the tunnel."

Sheila

I met Sheila, who was 28 years old, after she had had several cycles of IVF without success and had finally received a diagnosis of a rare chromosomal abnormality (after trying to become pregnant for three years). She came to see me after being referred by her reproductive endocrinologist (RE) when she had had several episodes of uncontrollable crying in the RE's office. While feeling both emotionally and financially challenged, Sheila, whose seven-year marriage to Kurt was in poor shape, was grimly gripping her options like a vise. She wanted to move rapidly ahead and do IVF with a donor egg, find a surrogate, and do a home study for adoption.

Sheila's only defense against deep despair and feelings of annihilation of her identity as a woman was to keep moving forward, at breakneck speed, without stopping to take a breath. My initial reaction to hearing about her plans to adopt, and the utter lack of any evidence of any kind of reflection about this process, was one of panic. I, too, felt spurred on to action and an urgent pressure to grab hold of Sheila, pin her down and "make her see" that all this was too soon, that she was not thinking it through, that her marriage was in trouble (in fact, she was dangerously close to starting an affair), and that she was not ready to adopt. As she proceeded in sessions to talk more and more about anything *but* the infertility or the adoption, and took a flight into a new social world, new friends, and a new romantic interest, I increasingly found myself becoming some kind of judge and jury, a hounding conscience, a voice of morality.

I worried about the child to be adopted and had fantasies of a child arriving and being forgotten and abandoned by Sheila. My concerns began to drown out my capacity to stay present with Sheila while she was with me, as I felt myself drift off into a kind of reverie of my own while I was with her. As I gradually became aware of what I was feeling, and what was happening between *us*, I was able to say, "You know, Sheila, I can't stop feeling like a judge and jury with you. What do you make of that?"

Sheila visibly relaxed and began to connect with her feelings about trying to have a child. She talked about her fears of being "sinful." Gradually, Sheila and I found a way to begin to talk about her experiences and her pain. She told me that, besides feeling "bad" at her core for being the infertile person in the couple, the very idea of using assisted reproductive medicine, which conflicted with her strong religious family values, felt like a sin. She went on to talk about her fear of rejection by her stern, authoritarian father, whom she was convinced would reject all reproductive options other than "natural" ones as "against God's wishes." She described experiences when she had felt abandoned by him when she was not behaving according to his strict standards. As she was growing up, the only means she had of escaping the strong, judgmental dictates of her father was to escape into worlds of fantasy and to "be bad," as she embraced the immoral crowd that he so deplored. This identification was overdetermined, as there was a split in her family between Sheila and her older sister, with whom she was still very competitive. Her sister had always been the "good daughter" while they were growing up, by virtue of her academic and athletic achievements, and today, by virtue of her financial security and, most of all her fertility (her sister had three sons).

The example of Sheila demonstrates the urgency that drives many women (and some men) experiencing infertility to move toward adoption as a way to *keep moving*, to get to the goal of having a child, without feeling the pain and despair along the way. For therapists, this example shows the familiar experience of identification with important figures in the patient's past, as well as the felt experience of the disowned "hounding affects" from which Sheila was fleeing. This clinical example illustrates the way that each person's individual psychodynamics interacts with infertility and adoption. For example, the experience of competition with her sister intersected with Sheila's feelings about the birth mother, while her feelings of badness were projected onto the unborn adopted child.

This vignette also illustrates the presence of powerful and familiar concerns that typically arise when encountering adoption, as my fantasy of the adopted child arriving and being forgotten and abandoned introduces the adoption triad: birth mother/father, adoptive parents, and adopted child. Contained in my fantasy are concerns for the (abandoned) child, the rejecting/neglecting mother, as well as an implied "rescuing mother" figure. In my experience, these are all common elements that come up when encountering adoption. These elements can either interfere, or be used productively, when recognized and reflected upon by the therapist.

WHEN TO ENCOURAGE ADOPTION EXPLORATION?

Sometimes the therapist needs to help the patient move on from medical treatments to looking at other options, including adoption. Doing so is very difficult when one considers that each person's threshold for pain is different, and when one tries to be respectful of the person's freedom to make his or her own choices. How do you know when to intervene? Sometimes I intervene when I feel that the person is being self-destructive, and sometimes I do so when I feel great pain at hearing what the patient is tolerating. This is what happened with Rebecca.

Rebecca

I met Rebecca when she was almost 42 years old and had been on her "infertility journey" for over four years. Like so many other women, Rebecca had "been through the mill." She had endured intrusive procedures and surgeries for multiple fertility problems, including blocked tubes, fibroids, and reduced ovarian reserve. She had been through two miscarriages, an ectopic ("tubal") pregnancy, several surgeries, and several cycles of IVF, the most recent of which had been cancelled because she was not producing enough eggs. A "trooper," Rebecca bravely soldiered on, obediently following instructions to a T, barely complaining, and researching website after website to educate herself about all the medical details she could find. Her husband was a faint character to me.

What I felt most exposed to, and what I was most aware of in sessions, was Rebecca's *insides*. As she spoke of procedure after procedure, I felt my body empathize (Aron and Anderson, 1998; LaBarre, 2001) with hers and found myself visualizing red flesh and the sore interior of her body. As she spoke of new protocols, new procedures, I found myself increasingly preoccupied with the *inside* of her body. I felt a silent horror and a great helplessness, and I was concerned about what to do with these feelings. I considered disclosing them to her, but I was concerned that to do so would be burdensome and intrusive and would make her feel even more shame. I also felt too guilty in sessions to inquire about her past or to explore the meanings of her experiences with her, as I would usually do; I felt that I would be avoiding her present pain if I did. I became curious about this hesitance, as well as the guilt and my preoccupation with hot, red flesh. I was also curious about my use of the word "brave" and the expression "soldiered on." I forced myself to explore further but felt as though I were betraying her needs as I did so. What I discovered was that Rebecca had a particularly sadistic father, whom she had always tried to placate by conforming to his rigid, almost military, routines. He had frequently demanded that his family endure what most would consider abusive treatment, both verbally and by his cruel and harsh "spankings." This discovery enabled me to consider with Rebecca if, in fact, she had been trying to please the doctor in the same way that she had felt bound to keep her father "happy." I asked what she thought would happen if she "disobeyed"; we started to see how anxious this idea made her and how she felt an absence of freedom in this area. I also recommended, quite strongly, that she start to explore other options, including adoption, while simultaneously I recognized with her the concern that I, too, must inevitably fall into the trap of also "telling her what to do." We started to talk about this. She also started to explore other options, and, for the first time in four years, "took some time off" from her infertility treatments to broaden her life and do something else. This shift produced a great softness and self-acceptance in her, and she proceeded to explore adoption and also egg donation.

PREMATURE MOVE TO ADOPTION

Sometimes people take to adoption like "a duck to water." Usually this makes me feel nervous, unless there is some historical reason why adoption would come so naturally. But when someone who has previously been uncomfortable with the idea of adoption suddenly starts talking about it in only positive or idealized terms, I often either feel unbelieving or have a great concern. Thus I experience the denial and fears that have been expelled or disowned by the people considering adoption. This can happen for many different reasons: often it is because adoption is too painful to explore, in which case I try to encourage the adopters to look more deeply beneath the surface, at least to locate their ambivalence. Sometimes other intrapersonal factors contribute to the inaccessibility of ambivalence, which happened with Susan and Thomas.

Susan and Thomas

Susan and Thomas were a devoted couple in their late 30s, quite religious, and very involved in their families and their community. They were both high achievers, and both depended on being active as a major part of their defensive structure. This approach had stood both of them in good stead in the past, as they each had triumphed over adversity by working hard and taking action. But this approach no longer worked in the area of infertility, with which they had struggled for more than three years when I met them. By this time they had endured various procedures, most of which were experienced as particularly noxious by Susan, who had been a "natural health food fanatic" prior to infertility and "had rarely even used an aspirin before." They each had difficulty feeling helpless and out of control and preferred to talk about family problems (Susan) and statistical probabilities (Thomas) during sessions, instead of difficult feelings.

They let me know at the beginning of our work together that they would be parents "no matter what" and that, if all else failed, they would "turn to adoption." They did not discuss this option for quite some time until it became evident that Susan could not use her own eggs owing to premature ovarian failure. At this time, they moved quickly "into adoption gear." Thomas, who had previously expressed great concern about the idea of adoption, suddenly had a change of heart. "It's like I finally woke up. One day adoption was not something I wanted to do, and the next day it suddenly became OK."

I felt a familiar sense of dread. I did not believe him. I was waiting for the other shoe to drop. *I*, not *he*, was in touch with his denial and their fears.

Susan, for her part, spent time telling me in detail that it was not a big adjustment. "I've always liked the idea of adoption. I knew a girl once who was adopted, and she turned out all right. I think I would be totally OK with it."

As I looked at this couple, they had smiles on their faces, which seemed rather "stuck," and the whole scenario felt "fake" or forced. And yet for some time I had difficulty gaining access to their ambivalence and fears about adoption. Finally, I was able to "open things up" after I talked about what I knew about them historically. Focusing here on Susan, I said, "You know, Susan, I've been thinking about how you've always been so very *good* in your life. You have been the responsible and reliable daughter, the one caring for your aging parents." (She agreed.) I continued, "Well, I wondered if part of this quick shift toward adoption is because you feel you "have to be good" here too, that you have to adopt, because you believe it is the right thing to do, to do what is expected of you, even if you'd rather try to consider egg donation."

Susan's whole face changed. She looked surprised and also guilty. She realized that she had not really allowed herself this "selfish" option, which would provide her with the longed-for opportunity to be pregnant, and that she had been trying to please family members (and internalized figures). We then started to explore egg donation, as well as Susan's feelings of anger about being infertile. Shortly afterward, Thomas started to talk about his own fears about adoption, and Susan and he were able to feel their ambivalence. From there we started the real exploration of adoption and egg donation.

IN THE MIDDLE OF THE BRIDGE

The middle of the bridge is often the point at which adoption becomes more real, the decision to adopt is made, unrealistic expectations recede, and the dream of the perfect, biological, "fantasy" child begins to be relinquished. For others who have already made the decision, this becomes a time of choosing an approach or of changing a route to follow (many people who dive right into adoption end up changing their routes). The need to adopt a child as close as possible to the biological child that would have been becomes less important, and people begin to consider other options, such as older children or children from different racial or ethnic backgrounds. Likewise, the idea of open adoption becomes less frightening as people become better educated and learn the advantages that this option brings.

Interestingly, the choice of different approaches is always made for the same reason, "because I could have more control." The emphasis on control is not surprising, given how out of control people experiencing infertility feel, but that this answer is given for different routes and choices demonstrates, I believe, the interface between commonality and individual differences. For example, one couple may choose a domestic, independent adoption, because, "It gives us more control. This way we can have the baby immediately after he or she is born, when he or she is only three days old." Another couple may choose to adopt internationally because, "It gives us more control, because we don't have to worry about the birth mother changing her mind."

In my experience, if there were any single point in the journey that could be described as the most difficult, then it would have to be the middle of the bridge. There are many potential areas of difficulty and many have to do with decision making. For some people, the difficulty is that they have not yet decided to adopt; others, who have been pursuing adoption for some time, no longer feel that they are making any headway with deciding which route to take. Many find this area of decision making more difficult than when they were involved in infertility treatments. Many avoid making decisions to try to avoid the inevitable loss that accompanies the decision. I find that ambivalence is usually greatest before a decision is made.

In fact, the *deliberateness* of adoption, the way it involves so many choices and decisions, which often feel like recommitments by adopters, creates many opportunities for people to lose momentum, for intercouple conflicts to reoccur, and for the process to become derailed. As in anything else, people carry themselves with them on the journey, and those people who are active, rather than passive, are more likely to continue their forward momentum.

The middle of the journey is often a time when adoption comes into focus, when it becomes more real, and when some people may decide adoption is not for them. This is not to say that the journey has been for nothing; the journey always provides a greater clarity, which enables people to move ahead, satisfied that they are clearer about their needs and goals than before. For those who move toward third-party-assisted reproduction, there is an added appreciation of the similarities between that and adoption, and always a greater appreciation of the needs and interests of the child. Here are some examples of people at the middle of the bridge.

Angela and Robert: Stuck Like Glue

Some people feel that they are in a no man's land, where they cannot proceed and yet they cannot turn back either. For couples who have run out of time, the issues of being stuck, of resistance to moving forward are overdetermined and compounded by their original resistance to becoming parents in the first place. This is what happened with Angela and Robert.

Angela and Robert, a professional couple in their late 40s, came to see me for help with their difficulties with moving forward in any direction toward having a child. The couple had married later in life, and, for most of their 10-year marriage, they had been undecided about having children. Angela had recently been pursuing infertility treatments and was currently signed up with one program to do egg donation, while simultaneously investigating adoption. They simply could not agree on which way to turn.

Angela was frustrated. She described years of ambivalence when the couple had not been able to come to agreement; the result was that she was now too old to conceive with her own eggs. She blamed Robert for this delay and seemed to feel hopeless about their future. Robert, for his part, avoided all talk about infertility, adoption, egg donation, and even reproduction and focused all his energies instead, both inside and outside the sessions, on talking about his difficulties at work. (This is an example of how men and women often have different coping reactions to infertility; see Mazure and Greenfeld, 1989.)

The two seemed ensconced in a stuckness that seemed as thick as stodgy porridge. I had the impression that I had been turned to as some sort of last resort, and I felt a great pressure to enliven the atmosphere of the sessions and come up with some impossible, magical solution.

After some initial exploration, which quickly got derailed by Robert's persistent focus on his work, and as I gradually became more aware of my internal pressures, I was able to use my countertransference to empathize with Robert's resistance and with his internal world. We spent many sessions talking about his work and the ways in which he felt unappreciated by Angela. The deep internal pressures he felt and the need, "the last resort," to "do the impossible" or something very special (or magical?) plagued him at every turn. Gradually, Robert began to feel understood by me, and I was able to reach him, which created hope for Angela. The turning point was a dream, in which Robert was competing with Superman (a superhero who was himself adopted—a common figure in dreams about adoption) and always coming up short. The exploration of this dream helped all of us to understand the ways in which Robert carefully protected himself against deep, long-standing feelings of inadequacy about his masculinity by his compulsive focus on his work.

As the therapy progressed, Robert started to feel more competent, and, as this happened, he began to challenge Angela. I was able to help both of them see that he had a point and that in some ways his talents and achievements had been unappreciated by Angela. As his competency was recognized, Robert was able to acknowledge deep feelings of guilt for having held both of them back. We were able to understand the historical precedents for his reluctance to have a biological child (because of his fear of becoming his sadistic father) and his deep personal feelings of shame and inadequacy, and they started to embrace the idea of adoption.

As we proceeded, Angela was able to show her vulnerability, and they began to work as a team. With much more exploration of historical experiences on both sides, the couple began to move forward. They were able to explore adoption issues with great sensitivity. Robert contributed fully from his empathy towards the adopted child's possible future struggles, his own feelings of imperfection, and his dedication to using his own struggles to help their future child with any potential difficulties along the way. They proceeded steadily toward adoption.

This example illustrates the importance of meeting people where they stand, and using my understanding of resistance and countertransference to move the treatment forward: when I do not try to control what is happening, but instead trust the *process*, then movement starts to occur. This couple's resistance to moving forward had to do with "pockets" of unexplored tension between them related to Robert's relationship with his father and his fears of biological and genetic continuity. Once we were able to gain access to this area, and to understand it, the questions about adoption, parenthood, and the necessary decisions unfolded. If I had tried to *make* this couple talk about reproduction or adoption, I believe we would have had much more difficulty moving forward together.

COUPLE DISAGREEMENT

Couples have to make many decisions about infertility and adoption, and, while many rely on the authority and authorization of the medical doctor during infertility treatments, people exploring adoption often find themselves more "out of sync" with their partners than they have ever been before. Sometimes this lack of agreement carries significant historical individual meaning, as was the case with Janet and Lee.

Janet and Lee

Janet and Lee, a Caucasian couple in their early 40s, came to see me for help in deciding which route to take toward having a child. They both came from working-class families and had had their share of hardships in life: Lee had lost both parents in late adolescence, and Janet had lost her older sister (and only sibling) through suicide. They had been married for 18 months, during which, in order not to "waste time," they had been trying to conceive.

Their desire to have a biological child was cut short when Janet discovered that not only were her eggs too old, but also she was perimenopausal. The reproductive endocrinologist they had consulted told them, "You won't conceive with your own eggs. You'll have to change a gamete." (This approach is not atypical of doctors working within the medical model, where egg donation is regarded as another medical treatment.) Lee could not get over his anger and sense of betrayal, which he directed at the doctor's delivery of the news: "What's it got to do with him? I'd like to kick him in his gametes!"

Janet blamed herself "for not knowing better." The shock of realizing that "the clock had stopped" without her knowing it was compounded by the shock and added loss of finding out that she was perimenopausal. That they had started to try to conceive as soon as they were married was forgotten, as both engaged in self-recrimination and attempts at undoing. They initially told me that they wanted help in deciding on whether to use a donor egg or to adopt. They complained of feeling stuck and at odds with each other for the first time. Neither felt particularly clear about a preferred route; they were most aware of deep feelings of loss and betrayal (Lee by "the medical establishment," Janet by her body and herself).

It became clear early on that neither was attracted to the idea of using a donor egg. Both felt that this route presented too much of a risk of their using up their slim financial resources. They were also uncomfortable with the idea. Lee said, "There's something unnatural about it. If you're going to change the egg, it's just the same as adoption anyway, so why not just go ahead and adopt?"

They both thought that the odds of having a child were much better through the adoption route. We were able to explore their feelings about the infertility and connect their losses with their pasts. But explore as we might, they could not agree on the path to take toward adoption. Lee wanted to do an independent, domestic adoption of a Caucasian infant, and Janet wanted to do an international adoption of a child from a different racial background. Both gave the same reason for their choices: they wanted to be sure that the child had been freely given up. Lee challenged how such a guarantee would be possible in an international adoption. "How would you know whether or not the child had been stolen?" Janet was concerned that a domestic birth mother would feel coerced.

Janet was also very fearful of doing an independent adoption; she would be expected to talk with birth mothers (adoption lawyers encourage women to talk to the birth mothers who answer advertisements about adoption). She felt uneasy at the idea of their "giving me their child, as if I would be persuading them."

I found it a challenge to work with this couple, partly due to Lee's anger and suspiciousness of me as a representative of the "establishment." I found myself feeling annoyed with him, and I often felt misunderstood and maligned. I was, however, able to use this countertransferential experience to engage Lee in a consideration of the nontraditional aspects of becoming an adoptive family, and what started out as appearing oppositional became, in my opinion, an engagement in a useful challenge of traditional ideas of parenting and family, for Lee was not afraid to take an unconventional approach to parenting. Unusual in my experience (usually it was the woman who moved first), Lee was the first in this couple to move sharply forward to embrace adoption as his chosen route. He identified strongly with both the possibility of being raised by someone other than one's biological parents (he himself had been raised by a distant aunt when his parents died) as well as the possibility of acknowledging two sets of parents (which was, again, similar to his own experience). He became frustrated with Janet for holding back. As he became more proactive, Janet got more depressed: not only did she blame herself for being the one who "caused the (infertility) problem," but now she felt even worse because she was causing another kind of problem by not being able to move ahead. Lee, who is a person of action, wanted, "to get on with it already." We seemed to be at a standstill.

The shift came after Janet came to a session alone one day. I asked about her fears of the birth mother's being pressured "to give the baby up to us." I was aware of her feelings of guilt. I was also remembering her sister's suicide, and I was thinking of survivor guilt. As we explored the possible meanings of the idea of the birth mother being pressured to "give the baby up," not only did Janet come to recognize how deeply she felt responsible for her sister's death, but also she was able to connect her feelings of guilt for the birth mother's loss with her feelings of guilt about her sister's death. She did not want "to cause pain or take something that was not mine" (she felt she had taken over her older sister's position in the family). (Here, adoption was regarded as stealing, and loss of infertility was perhaps seen as being robbed.) She was also able to see that she was interested in adopting a child from a different racial background because she felt she "did not deserve" what she really wanted, a white child. Not long after this session, Janet and Lee made a decision to adopt a white child through a reputable private agency. They intended to do an open adoption, in which they would try to diminish the sense of loss of all three participants (themselves, their child, and the birth mother/parents) and they could also be assured that the birth mother/parents were being treated fairly.

This example illustrates how historical and intrapersonal issues interact with adoption to bring additional layers of meaning to the adoption process. While the therapist is negotiating agreement between couples, it is important to elucidate, where appropriate, the individual meanings of adoption, to help the couple understand each other, and proceed to a plan that is acceptable to both members of the couple. This particular treatment, and my empathy with Robert's oppositional feelings toward authorities aroused my own ambivalent feelings about authority. I believe that some professionals and experts in the field of adoption often end up becoming an intrusive authoritarian presence, not infrequently disempowering people and making it less likely that they will feel confident about their own ability to make decisions for themselves. While I believe that all professionals do, to some degree, become authorities with their patients, and that to some degree this is unavoidable, I also believe that what promotes change is the encouragement of exploration and the engagement of curiosity, rather than the imposition of authority.

THE PATH OF MOST RESISTANCE: NARCISSISM

To move from the middle to the end of the bridge, adopters need to become more comfortable with their feelings about their infertility, although a complete resolution is neither necessary nor possible. This exploration may reactivate a narcissistic coping style (Rosen, 2002) from the experiences of infertility, where self- and other-perceptions are flattened and reduced. This seemed to be the case with Celia and Richard.

Celia and Richard

I met Celia and Richard after they had moved from infertility toward adoption for the second time after five years of infertility treatment. Their previous foray into adoption followed a painful miscarriage and led to the decision to try donor egg first. When this donor egg IVF did not work, Celia experienced such emotional pain that the couple decided to end infertility treatment once and for all and move back to adoption.

When I met them, this highly attractive, highly successful professional couple looked depressed, beaten down, and resigned. While Celia talked with grim determination about this "second best" choice, Richard seemed preoccupied and passive and kept looking at his watch. Both seemed to feel great shame that they had been unable to conceive (a combination of male factor and advanced female age), and both felt guilty that they had not tried earlier in their 15-year marriage. When I met them, they had done everything toward an independent adoption except place advertisements in newspapers for adoption. Although they both really seemed to want a child and had gone to great lengths to pursue both paths, they still wondered if they should adopt or remain child free. They had been struggling in this area for some time, and both were exhausted and emotionally drained.

Of the two, Celia seemed to feel more like a failure. When I asked her how she felt about adoption, she strongly implied that she thought adoption and adoptive mothering were inferior. When I pointed out this seeming implication to her, she seemed irritated, as though I were wasting her time by "going through the motions," when all along she "knew the truth." She appeared impatient when I tried to help them explore what it would be like to become an adoptive family. Although Richard appeared to welcome this question and became more engaged afterward, Celia stiffened and responded, "I don't have a problem with adoption. It wouldn't make a difference to me. It's just the rest of the world's reactions and prejudices that I'm worried about."

Celia, a bright, attractive woman who looked much younger than her years, and Richard, also an attractive man, were highly successful in all other areas of their lives. Both had reached the top of their chosen professions. They had a lovely apartment and a lively social life. They enjoyed eating out, going to the theater regularly, and taking creative and exotic vacations. In fact, I found myself feeling some envy of their lives, even as I felt their infertility pain, which was greatly increased by their difficulty making a "final decision."

The envy I felt was an important key for me. Although envy is common in infertility, which greatly exaggerates this feeling in most women and some men, I was feeling more envy than I usually do, and I became curious. Of the two, Celia was the most vocal about her ambivalence, and so it was on her that I mainly focused my attention. I knew that Celia was very competitive and motivated by "success"; I also knew she struggled with negative feelings about adoption, which she largely projected onto the adopted child, expecting gratitude or reward, rather than recognizing a need to parent. "I would never be able to accept a child telling me I wasn't its 'real mother,' not after I'd gone to all that trouble!" (Here, adoption is seen as reparation for Celia's badly damaged sense of self, and the adopted child is seen as an object or commodity.)

I thought about the birth mother, whom Celia rarely mentioned. I remembered Celia's rivalry with her sister, who had four healthy, biological children, and I felt the competition between us in sessions. I wondered aloud how Celia and Richard would need to change their lives if they were to proceed toward adoption. I asked what stopped them from proceeding. I mused about how would their "life narrative" need to change. Celia was curious; she told me that, until that point, she had considered that their "narrative," their "story," was already set in stone: "Infertility was the one area in my life that I failed at. I waited too long. What was I thinking?"

I asked Celia what adopting would mean to her, and she immediately said, "Failure. That I did it to myself, that I waited too long, that I missed the boat." I then asked her if *that* was what was holding her back; in other words, if the idea of adoption felt like an *acknowledgment of defeat*, of seeing her past decisions and medical treatments as a *failure*. She became curious. We spent some time talking about what had kept her from seeking out parenthood earlier, and she explained that she, like many women, had thought that she was comfortable being childless right up until she realized that time was running out, at which point she and Richard changed their minds. As she remembered and talked about the past, she began to feel more accepting and less critical of herself (and of Richard, whom she blamed for not pushing her to become a mother earlier).

We also looked at how her competitiveness and narcissistic drive towards perfection kept her from "taking the plunge," how these protected her from coming into contact with difficult feelings, and how these made it hard for her to reflect on the imperfections of the adopted child, her own imperfections, and the presence of a second mother who was "more perfect" because she was fertile (the birth mother). As we talked, Celia and Richard came to grieve, but also to feel more accepting, Celia, of herself and also of each of them as a couple, as they learned to see that they could accept that they "were not ready" earlier. They were then able to embrace adoption as "an imperfect solution for imperfect people in an imperfect world."

AT THE END OF THE BRIDGE

By the time people reach the end of the bridge, each person will be changed, for by now adoption is *real* and the definition of *being a family* has been expanded. Most people have already decided to adopt and have been actively pursuing this option, while others may need a clear plan to return back across the bridge for more medical treatments, often of limited treatment trials (usually one), before possibly returning to adoption. Many have decided to end medical treatment and have been grieving the loss of their biological child. Some have moved away in other directions, toward alternative paths to family building, while still others have decided to remain child free, either actively or by slipping into childlessness through passivity. Some people move toward adoption choices that they previously could not have imagined, such as international or open adoption.

However, not all the issues regarding adoption are settled, far from it. For it is now widely believed that the transition to an integrated acceptance of adoption as a welcome family-building option takes time and is an ongoing process over the family's lifetime, in much the same way as infertility is now considered to be a lifelong, rather than a discrete process (Brodzinsky, Schechter, and Marantz Hening, 1992; Brodzinsky, 1997). But by the time people are close to the end of the bridge, they are closer to letting go of the previously cherished idea and goal of biological and genetic continuity, of having the much-fantasized-about "(biological) child of our own," and of being part of the world of people who reproduce in the usual way. Some are beginning to see that there is more than one way to have a child "of their own," that they can embrace unexpected options. People begin to see some of the advantages of nonbiological connectedness: "I've been thinking that it will be easier to raise this child to let him or her be who he or she is, without imposing my own expectations, which I think I would do if the child were mine biologically."

People begin to feel a growing sense of hope and excitement and to look ahead to being parents, rather than being focused on adoption issues per se. This is a point where a sense of continuity begins to grow. For some, their world-view and existential experience of life has been affected, and the experience of being out of control may have become more of an acceptance of life's limits, as well as an appreciation for life's surprises. The past tends to be rewritten, and the phrase, "I've always wanted to adopt," is returned to in a new and different way, with more of a sense of integrating adoption with the past, rather than the rationalization it previously seemed. This is the beginning of a sense of belonging, of connectedness, bonding, and attachment. For adoptive families do connect in deep and powerful ways, other than biologically. Almost all adoptive parents talk about how they were "fated" to be parents to their (adopted) children (Kirk, 1964, 1981).

At this time, people begin to look at the future, both in terms of parenting issues and with a better understanding of the long-range impact of infertility. There is an opportunity here to help people begin to anticipate not only how infertility will retreat and reappear at typical junctures, such as when their adopted children become fertile, a time that can remind infertile adoptive parents of their own infertility, but also of parenting areas that may be difficult to navigate, such as issues of separation, autonomy, and individuation, and periods of potential difficulty such as adolescence. It is very important to help people feel their ambivalence and to accept ambivalence as normal (I find this is an area where adoptive parents, as well as people who have reproduced biologically after infertility, often have difficulty).

BRINGING FAMILY ON BOARD

While all prospective adoptive parents struggle with issues of disclosure, for some the decisions are more difficult than for others. Often there is the expectation of rejection, and the sharing of the decision to adopt can be difficult and painful. When the infertility treatments have not been disclosed to family members, adoption can make disclosure even more difficult.

Joan and John

I met with Joan and John when they were well into their adoption process. A private couple, Joan and John had moved to New York City partly in an attempt to escape their "small-town" pasts and to reinvent themselves. To a large degree, that is exactly what they had done, creating a life for themselves that was very different from that of each of their original families. Their distance from their families did not, in fact, appear to bother either of them until they decided to have a child, at which point Joan felt a longing for a greater closeness with her mother and sisters. Their (male factor) infertility was painful, and they chose not to share this information with their families so as to protect John from feelings of shame. After three years of trying to conceive, they decided to adopt. They were doing an independent adoption, things had moved along more quickly than they had expected, and they had a "situation" (a pregnant woman who had answered their advertisements for a baby). They were discussing with her adopting her unborn child, and yet they still had not yet told either family. They wanted my help with this.

Joan was annoyed that John had "not allowed" her to tell her family what was going on: "If only we'd told them before, all this would have been so much easier." John explained, "I didn't see the point before. They didn't need to know, and then we didn't know if we would even have children at all. And now this adoption has moved so quickly, we've barely had time to think."

As we explored what had held them back, it became clear that it was a combination of John's shame and his fear that his father would reject their adopted child that held them back. Joan did not want to "lie" to her family, by letting them think that the infertility was "her problem," and she did not want to protect John anymore. This was the issue we focused on first, with an exploration of Joan's pent-up anger from the inequity of the situation, her anger at John for refusing to consider sperm donation, and her anger that he had not recognized how his "selfish" demands for secrecy had made things difficult for her. For his part, John's deep feelings of shame made it difficult for him to talk about his infertility. As they communicated their individual pain, they were able to feel less distance from each other. I struggled with feeling overwhelmed and "not knowing which issue to face first." I felt swept up in something that was too powerful to direct or control, a resonance with the internal worlds of Joan and John, as well as the immediacy of the adoption situation. As all three of us discussed their difficult feelings toward each other, and toward their infertility, the reality of the possible imminent adoption pulled the focus back to the issues of disclosure.

John wanted to tell both families something vague on the telephone, without explaining why they had decided to adopt; Joan wanted to visit each family in person and "come clean." I encouraged John to explore why he was so reluctant to tell his family, and he was finally able to talk about the longstanding and constant humiliation he had received from his father and four brothers for being "like a sissy." He was concerned that he would be the object of scorn if they knew "I shoot blanks." The shame and humiliation was palpable, and I felt empathy for John and had difficulty connecting with Joan's feelings of anger and frustration. Joan seemed unmoved, and she and John continued to argue as the due date for the birth mother approached. I understood (and interpreted) that at least part of this conflictive exchange was a way of tolerating their anxiety about the approaching birth.

The issue of an "in person" visit to their parents (in distant parts of the country) became a moot point, as the possibility of parenthood fast approached, and they both needed to conserve their vacation time for parenthood. Finally, a week before the baby's due date, they called each family and, using two telephones, they shared their news with both families with as much enthusiasm as they could muster. Joan did more of the talking with John's family, and agreed that, with his family, at least, they would only share that they had "fertility problems" without going into any detail (their compromise was that she could tell selected people, such as her mother and sisters, as long as they kept it private). Two days later their baby was born, and they were swept up in parenthood. They told me later that John's father "came around as soon as he saw his new granddaughter, and now he is her greatest admirer."

Not all adoption stories have such a happy ending (or beginning), both in terms of the speed (most independent adoptions take a lot longer), success (some birth mothers change their minds, which is very painful for those hoping to adopt), and the disclosure. In my experience, all people who move from infertility to adoption struggle with issues of disclosure, whether or not they have previously disclosed their infertility. The fears of rejection by close family members are yet another part of the fear of loss that pervades this experience. Many reluctant family members (but not all) "come around" when they see the adopted child in person. I find it helpful to remind people who are adopting but who are afraid of others' reactions how far they have come and what they used to feel about adoption at the beginning of their journey. In fact, I believe that the concept of a journey is probably the single most useful idea and intervention, for it helps contextualize the process of change and development, as well as frame an understanding that others may be further behind in the process.

AFTER ADOPTION

Sometimes people move straight to adoption without considering the emotional impact of this move. The result is that they have a delayed reaction to infertility issues that can seriously affect their well-being and the integrity of their relationship with the adopted child.

Common issues include a withdrawal and (often unconscious) rejection of the adopted child, as grief issues either remain unresolved or are triggered in a delayed reaction, which can significantly interfere with the parents' capacity to be present for their child and to face the many ongoing challenges of parenting.

WHEN THE PATIENT IS ADOPTED

Because the trend toward openness in adoption that is currently influencing adoptive parenting has only emerged during the past 20 years, it is likely that many adoptees have been raised with relatively little discussion of their adoption and what it means either to them or to their families. For many adoptees, issues of adoption may surface in full force at important junctures, perhaps the most significant of which is when they decide to become parents; this coming into contact with adoption issues is intensified when infertility occurs. Sometimes the emergence of strong feelings about adoption is quite unexpected.

Kyra

Kyra was a pleasant, attractive, successful achiever who had solid relationships with her husband, family, and friends and a successful career. The oldest daughter (and only adopted child) in a family of four children (one brother and two sisters), Kyra was her father's favorite and was respected and "adored" by her younger siblings. Everything seemed to be almost perfect in her life. The only apparent ripple was her longstanding infertility. Kyra reacted to her infertility with some depression but was not derailed by it or by the many difficult and intrusive procedures she had endured in her infertility treatment. Due to a long history of endometriosis, Kyra often endured pain and had had some surgeries, as well as one ectopic pregnancy, which led to the loss of one of her fallopian tubes. She became pregnant during her third IVF cycle, and her immediate joy was palpable. It was during the early stages of her pregnancy, as the pregnancy became more real, that Kyra first started to have feelings about having been adopted.

No one was more surprised than Kyra that she started to become preoccupied with her birth parents, and particularly with her birth father. During this time, she talked only with her husband and with me about this preoccupation. She felt some guilt about talking about it at all, for she felt that she was being disloyal to her adoptive family and particularly to her adoptive mother, with whom she had a very close relationship. She told me she also disliked keeping secrets, especially from her adoptive mother. She also seemed to be uncomfortable discussing her relationship with her adoptive mother with me as well, and said she felt it was disloyal. I understood this to be possibly a remnant of the family system, in which the birth mother was too threatening to be acknowledged. Kyra gradually, in her very distinctive cautious, careful, and deliberate way, started to put her feelings into words: "I can't believe I am feeling this way. I've never really thought about this before, and I just can't stop thinking about it. Now that I'm becoming a parent, I think about being adopted all the time. I couldn't possibly think of giving my baby up."

Although Kyra rarely mentioned her birth mother, she spoke of feeling guilty that she was pregnant, whereas other women experiencing infertility were not. She said, "I feel guilty that I was chosen." As we discussed this, she told me that she felt she had been given preferential treatment in her family, that her parents had always told her that she was "special" because she was "chosen." Gradually, I started to feel impatient with Kyra. I felt annoyed that she seemed to avoid talking about her birth mother. I felt annoyed that she was so protective of her adoptive mother. I started to feel annoyed that she was so "good." I started to feel *guilty* about being so annoyed. Because Kyra's pregnancy was high risk, and because I felt a need to be cautious, I did not work with her *explicitly* about my reactions during this time. Instead, consistent with my belief in the power of unconscious communication in the therapeutic dyad, I did more *internal* work, by recognizing my experiences with her and trying to reflect on and understand their possible meanings for her internal experience, her feelings about her adoption, and, in particular, her split-off anger.

I hypothesized that she had indeed felt a press to be "good," which was related partly to her experience of being "chosen," and that some of her feelings of guilt had to do with the "specialness" this experience afforded her in her family and the way her father openly favored her over her siblings. I wondered if she felt she had betrayed her adoptive mother by moving from infertility (a shared experience) to the biological and genetic continuity and link with her birth mother. I also considered her guilt toward her "fellow infertility sisters" at the clinic as reflective of aspects of the adoption triad: the adoptive mother's guilt toward the birth mother for having her child, and her envy of the birth mother's ability to bear a child, while she, the infertile adoptive mother, cannot.

I supported Kyra. I did not push her to explore the conspicuously absent birth mother. I felt that she would proceed when she was ready. When I last saw her, she was close to term, had met with her birth father, and had asked him about her birth mother, whom she was thinking of contacting. She shared this information with her family, including her mother, and they were all very support-ive. She looked glowing and had a wider range of affect. She did become irritable at times and appeared infinitely more human, while I, in my countertransference, felt much less irritated.

Looking back, I believe that my ability to trust myself and fol-low her lead was quite helpful to Kyra, who benefited from my "containment" as she made her way, at her own speed and in her own time. I believe that I "held" some of the more difficult feel-ings that she was so well defended against until she was feeling more certain of the viability of her pregnancy and could feel them herself. I think that being preoccupied with the birth father was easier for her than looking at her more charged feeling toward the birth mother. I think that the need to "keep mothers apart" was a longstanding one in her life.

EMBRYO ADOPTION AND THIRD-PARTY REPRODUCTION

This chapter would be incomplete without at least a brief acknowl-edgment of the common ground between traditional adoption and embryo adoption (also called embryo donation) and the use of donor gametes. Embryo adoption refers to the *social* sense of adop-tion, rather than the legal one, where adoption happens at the time of embryo transfer. Embryo adoption encompasses two different routes of using both a sperm and an egg that are not genetically related to the couple or individual who will gestate the embryo and parent the resulting child: the first is through a "donated" embryo (often donated by the genetic parents after they have already built their family and no longer need the embryo), and the second is through embryo creation, when the egg and sperm are intention-ally created for the purpose of transferring to the infertile person or couple. Donor gametes are either eggs or sperm that are not genetically related to the social parents. Many refer to these options as either prenatal adoption or preimplantation adoption (in the case of embryo adoption) or part or half-adoptions (in the case of the use of donor gametes).

There are many reasons for choosing these options. Embryo adoption offers the individual or couple privacy, the opportunity to experience pregnancy, the guarantee of known paternity (often not possible in adoption), and a greater sense of in-utero control and may offer decreased costs. Donor gametes offer privacy, the opportunity to experience pregnancy, and the opportunity for one parent to be genetically related to the child.

At the present time, many people who avail themselves of these options hear about them in a medical context, where there is often insufficient consideration of the psychosocial issues involved. Many mental health professionals see the parallels between the history of adoption and the current early beginnings of these new methods, and they believe and expect that the children born by these methods, as well as other third-party parenting options (surrogacy and gestational carriers), will have future, long-range issues similar to those discovered in the adoption triad. At present, there is no consensus on this issue, although there is ongoing debate, and comparisons are being made between adoption and third-party reproduction (see Cooper and Glazer, 1998; Freundlich, 2001).

These family-building routes share many of the same issues with adoption, such as questions of the importance of genetic history, issues of disclosure, and issues of belonging and connectedness. While some mental health professionals argue that the experience of gestating a child will help prevent some of the difficulties of adoptees, and even that children made this way should be protected from knowing how they were created, others argue that the importance of genetics will have a similar impact on the formation of the identity of people who are created this way and that those people have the right to know about their origins.

While being respectful of the rights of people considering these options to choose their own personal paths, I try to help the people I work with to consider the future effect of their decisions on their children, and I use parallels with adoption to illustrate these points. I have found that people who have explored traditional adoption and who then proceed toward one of these third-party options have an increased appreciation for the child as an individual, whose interests and needs are separate and distinct from those of the parent.

SUMMARY

People move from infertility to adoption in common and individual ways, through grief over the lost biological child, through understanding the differences in adoption, to embracing a new identity as adoptive parents who bond and attach through nonbiological pathways. The metaphor of the bridge and the idea of a journey both powerfully convey the developmental process of change involved in moving through infertility toward adoption (and other options). Any approach to working with people struggling with infertility and moving toward adoption has to be an integrated one that considers both people and adoption as complex. For just as all people are different, so are all adoptions different also. There is no "one size fits all" approach to adoption: adoptions are as different as the people in them, and there is no single "adoptive family template."

In my opinion, the recent changes in adoption and the development of third-party parenting options demonstrate a need for new models of development, with a greater recognition of and appreciation for the significance and impact of the triadic nature of these forms of parenting. For there is a dearth of theories and research that integrate adoption and other third-party methods of reproduction, as most models of personality and theories of child development are based on children who are biologically and genetically related to their parents and then superimposed on adoptive families and families built through other, nontraditional methods, rather than incorporating or being generated by these variations in family building.

People experiencing infertility who move toward adoption often need help in this transition to help them process and work through difficult feelings, thoughts, fears, myths, and ideas. They need help in deciding whether or not adoption is right for them, and they often need help to learn *how* to make decisions, which they can then carry forward into their lives. This ability for people to become empowered to discover what choices and decisions are right for them, and to rely and depend on their own judgment, is especially important for adoptive parents, for I believe that one of the central challenges for adoptive parenting is the tremendous *uncertainty* that is created by not knowing which issues are and which are not adoption related. The need to be mindful of how adoption is both ever-present and yet also alternately either in the foreground or the background of an individual's or a family's experience demands a sensitivity that adoptive parents may first learn from working with a mental health professional on their journey from infertility to adoption. In this journey, exploring is valued and empowering and leads to a greater capacity for reflection and the consideration of multiple perspectives (which is essential in adoptive parenting).

As therapists working with infertility and adoption, we are in a unique and powerful position to help people negotiate the fundamental and primitively central area of family building, as people adjust to their limits and embrace new and unexpected paths and options. I believe that one of the most treasured resources is our countertransference, which is informed by our understanding and awareness of ourselves and allows us access to the areas of greatest tension in the treatment, providing us with much of the necessary leverage to help our patients. In closing, I would like to end on a dialectical note of balance: if we consider that much of life is experienced as tensions between equidistant, opposing poles of experience, then we must consider not only the losses of adoption but also the *gains*, not only how people are lost in adoption, but also how they are *found*.

REFERENCES

Aron, L. & Anderson, F. S., eds. (1998), *Relational Perspectives on the Body*. Hillsdale, NJ: The Analytic Press.

Brodzinsky, D. M. (1997), Infertility and adoption adjustment: Considerations and clinical issues. In: *Infertility: Psychological Issues and Counseling Strategies*, ed. S. A. Leiblum. New York: Wiley, pp. 246–262.

———— Schechter, M. D. & Marantz Henig, R. (1992), *Being Adopted*. New York: Doubleday.

Cooper, S. L. & Glazer, E. S. (1998), *Choosing Assisted Reproduction*. Indianapolis, IN: Perspectives Press.

Freundlich, M. (2001), *Adoption and Ethics: Adoption and Assisted Reproduction.* Washington, DC: Child Welfare League of America.

Goldfarb, J. M., Rosenthal, M. B. & Utian, W. H. (1985), Impact of psychological factors in the care of the infertile couple. *Seminar Reprod. Endocrinol.*, 3:97.

Johnston, P. I. (1992), *Adopting After Infertility.* Indianapolis, IN: Perspectives Press.

Kirk, H. D. (1964), *Shared Fate.* New York: Free Press.

———— (1981), *Adoptive Kinship: A Modern Institution in Need of Reform.* Toronto, Can.: Butterworth.

LaBarre, F. (2001), *On Moving and Being Moved: Nonverbal Behavior in Clinical Practice.* Hillsdale, NJ: The Analytic Press.

Mazure, C. M. & Greenfeld, D. A. (1989), Psychological studies of in vitro fertilization/embryo transfer recipients. *J. in Vitro Fertilization & Embryo Transfer*, 6:242–256.

Melina, L. R. (1998), *Raising Adopted Children.* New York: HarperCollins.

Rosen, A. (2002), Binewski's family: A primer for the psychoanalytic treatment of infertility patients. *Contemp. Psychoanal.*, 38:345–370.

Winnicott, D. W. (1971), *Playing and Reality.* London: Tavistock.

Part III

Special Circumstances, Special Treatment Challenges

8

TREATING SINGLE MOTHERS BY CHOICE

Elizabeth A. Grill

CHILDREN GROWING UP WITHOUT FATHERS ARE MORE
LIKELY TO FAIL AT SCHOOL OR TO DROP OUT, ENGAGE IN
EARLY SEXUAL ACTIVITY, DEVELOP DRUG AND ALCOHOL
PROBLEMS, AND EXPERIENCE OR PERPETRATE VIOLENCE.

—Wade F. Horn, Ph.D.,
President, National Fatherhood Initiative

PARENTING IS A JOB, IT REQUIRES CERTAIN SKILLS AND
THE MATURITY TO CARRY THEM OUT—IT IS NOT SOMETHING
THAT COMES WITH A MARRIAGE LICENSE OR MALE GENES.

—Jane Mattes, C.S.W.,
Founder and Director of Single Mothers by Choice

*A*ccording to the 2000 United States Census, the number
of single mothers increased between 1970 and 2000 from 3 million to 10 million. Contrary to common assumptions, of the one
in three babies born in the United States to unwed mothers, 60%
are born to women older than 30. Where once out-of-wedlock
births were a teenage epidemic, the latest figures show teenagers

to have had only a slight increase in birth rate, while the birth rate for unmarried women in their early 20s through mid-30s has soared.

Although divorce is still the most common way for women to become single mothers, more than 40% of today's single moms have never been married, a statistic suggesting a significant shift in societal attitudes. While it is not known exactly how many of these births are planned and intentional, it is true that increasing numbers of women are choosing single motherhood. The largest increases are among white women and college educated women, particularly those with professional and managerial jobs.

HISTORICAL OVERVIEW

Artificial insemination has provided an answer for women who want to become pregnant without a male partner. In such requests, where there is no known fertility problem, the use of the treatment is justified on social rather than on medical grounds (Baetens et al., 1995).

Published discussions of the possibility that single women might request donor insemination (DI) date back to the 1940s and express great concern and distaste (Kritchevsky, 1981). The notion of motherhood by choice has only recently been more widely recognized by doctors and other health professionals. While there is considerably less stigma attached to single parenthood now, however, some single women still face considerable resistance.

WHY DO WOMEN CHOOSE ARTIFICIAL INSEMINATION?

Single women who decide to become mothers must decide whether to adopt or proceed through a pregnancy. Increasingly, single women are seeking artificial insemination by donors for many reasons. In a study by Leiblum, Palmor, and Spector (1995), 70% of the women reported four factors that had prompted them to begin DI treatment: (1) they feel secure in their employment; (2) they had worked through parenting issues for themselves; (3) they felt that time was passing; and (4) they felt that they had sufficient social support. All the women planned to disclose to the children the facts of their conception, but they were not always sure how and when to do so.

In several other studies (McCartney, 1985; Fidell and Marik, 1989; Baetens et al., 1995), the main reasons given by the respondents for choosing DI were as follows: (1) they did not have male friends whom they might ask to act as a donor for self-insemination or to be the child's natural father; (2) the women considered it immoral to mislead a man into fathering a child without his knowledge; (3) they did not wish to share responsibility for the child and wished to avoid problems with respect to any paternal rights of a biological father; and (4) because of the genetic and medical screening of donors, they thought there was less risk of sexually transmitted diseases or AIDS and of the baby's being born with congenital conditions.

In one investigation (McCartney, 1985), a high percentage of the single women were found to have a medical basis for their infertility. In another survey (Fidell and Marik, 1989), the advanced age of the applicants seemed to play an important part in their selecting treatment, referred to by the investigators as a "now or never" mentality. Consistent with the research in this area, Rosenthal (1990) described women in donor insemination programs at large medical centers as well educated, financially stable, and in their late 30s. They indicated that they wanted healthy, genetically related children before their "biological clocks" ran out. They described their relationships with others as sound. Their sexual orientations varied, as did their feminist or traditional views. They did not want brief, uninvolved sexual encounters, which some of them saw as exploitative. They did not want custody battles with known donors. They were generally more open about their plans than many heterosexual couples, who have sought artificial insemination using donors because of male infertility.

The earliest studies showed father absence to have negative outcomes with respect to children's cognitive, social, and emotional development (Herzog and Sudia, 1973; Strong and Schinfeld, 1984; McGuire and Alexander, 1985; Potter and Knaub, 1988; Baetens et al., 1995). Later investigations, which controlled for such factors as economic hardship and lower social class, found that the intellectual and educational level of children raised in female-headed families is not significantly different from that of children raised in two-parent families. Therefore, the absence of a father by itself is not adversely related to a child's social adjustment or intellectual ability (Broman, Nicholos, and Kennedy, 1975; Ferri, 1976; Cashion, 1982; McGurie and Alexander, 1985; Crockett, Eggebeen, and Hawkins, 1993).

Golombok, Tasker, and Murray (1997) found that children in father-absent households perceived themselves to be less cognitively and physically competent than their peers from father-present families. The researchers suggested that the presence of a father may be associated with a child's developing self-esteem. Other studies, however, found that girls from female-headed families are highly independent (Baruch, 1972), have high self-esteem (Cashion, 1982), and are highly achievement oriented (Hunt and Hunt, 1977).

MOTIVATIONS TO PARENT AS A SINGLE MOTHER

The motivations for pregnancy and bearing children are complex and multidetermined. The wish for a pregnancy is not always the same as that to bear and raise a child (Rosenthal, 1990). Although single women seeking donor insemination seem to be a very special group, they have some of the same conscious and unconscious motivations for wanting a pregnancy and a child as do married women. Many say that they always wanted to be mothers. Some desire a child to combat the fear of loneliness, to confirm their sexual identity and bodily capability, and to fulfill the expectations of their parents, society, and culture. Some women long for a child to rework the relationships with their own mothers. Some may be reacting to the loss of a relationship or of a parent. Some simply do not want to miss out on this major life experience (Nadelson, 1978; Jacob, 1999).

WHO IS THE SINGLE MOTHER BY CHOICE?

Bernard (1974) wrote about single women who wanted to adopt children and described them as "a new group" of women in their late 30s who were reared in large families. This new group were often professionals with good incomes who chose motherhood instead of wifehood. According to Bernard, they chose a child instead of a husband, although they did not abandon the idea of marriage. They had succeeded in their work roles and now wanted to try the mother role. Some single women choosing motherhood differed from traditional mothers in experiencing less guilt, having less self-sacrificing qualities, being less possessive, feeling that children did not owe them anything for their love, and being more androgynous in their values, more flexible and nonfuture oriented. Interestingly, they viewed marriage as more complex than motherhood.

Initially, research looking at families led by single mothers did not separate data regarding families of "single mothers by choice" from families of women who became single mothers in other ways (i.e., through accidental conception, rape, separation or divorce, or widowhood). One of the first attempts to categorize this heterogeneous group of unmarried women with children was made by Eiduson and colleagues (1982). In their research, they described three groups of single mothers. The first group of women were "unmarried mothers," very young mothers whose pregnancies were unwanted and who were financially dependent on relatives or social security. The second group were "post-hoc adapters," women who had not planned on getting pregnant but who managed to adapt to motherhood. The third group were "nest builders," slightly older women with successful careers and who had planned to get pregnant.

This last category, the "nest builders," is similar to unmarried mothers whose wish for motherhood supersedes their desire for a relationship and need for biological fathers to help raise the children. In a study by McCartney (1985) one single woman's statement was used to summarize the entire group: "Nothing is missing from my life. I just want to expand it."

Few studies (McCartney, 1985; Fidell and Marik, 1989) have explored this new group of women who are single by choice and who have sought assisted reproductive technologies to help fulfill their desire to have children. Overall, the women in these studies were financially stable and had a wide social network, which included men, and a family that approved of their choice and gave its full support.

In another study, by Leiblum, Palmer, and Spector (1995), of the 45 unmarried women who had undergone donor insemination, 28 were heterosexual, 14 were lesbian, 2 were bisexual, 1 was celibate.

There were few differences between the groups, except that the heterosexual women tended to be older. Other studies indicate that the decision to become a single mother took an average of four to five years. Single motherhood for these goal-directed women seemed a viable choice, and, overall, the women reported being happy with their decisions (Frank and Brackley, 1989).

There is some evidence that the average single mother by choice is, on the whole, better educated and holds a better job than the average American. Occupationally, they seem to hold higher status and better paid positions than women nationally. It is important to note, however, that single mothers by choice are not uniformly highly educated or middle class (Pakizegi, 1990). There are significant numbers of lower middle-class, low income, and unemployed women among them (Fox, 1980; Kornfein, 1985).

Some critics take issue with describing these women as single mothers by choice because for many of these women the decision to be a single mother was not a positive choice. In one investigation, almost all the women (91.49%) who applied for fertility treatment with DI noted that they would have preferred to have had a child within a stable heterosexual parent relationship rather than as a single person (Baetens et al., 1995). In fact, the literature suggests that most single women who choose to have a child hope to have a life partner later in their lives. Their age often forced them to decide between single motherhood or unwanted childlessness. According to Mattes (1997), "A single mother by choice is a woman who starts out raising her child without a partner. She may or may not marry later on, but at the outset, she is parenting alone" (p. 4).

The struggle to categorize this group of unmarried women with children has ensued for decades. The truth is that the single mother by choice of today has many faces. She is the young cancer survivor who freezes eggs prior to chemotherapy in order to preserve her chances of fertility later. She is the recently widowed young woman who wishes to have a child with her deceased husband's frozen sperm. She is the 44-year-old woman who never found "Mr. Right" to settle down or conceive with. She is the younger woman who wishes to concentrate on her career but wants to freeze her eggs to preserve her fertility for later. The following case studies introduce some of these women and the multifaceted set of issues that arise, as well as therapists' countertransferential reactions, due to the complex nature of working with this population.

COUNTERTRANSFERENCE AND FERTILITY PATIENTS

An increasing emphasis on the value of countertransference feelings has encouraged therapists to perceive uncomfortable feelings and thoughts as potentially precious handles to a patient's unconscious (Winnicott, 1949; Little, 1951; Racker, 1968; Kernberg, 1976). In this chapter, countertransference is defined as the total response to the patient, both conscious and unconscious (Tansey and Burke, 1995) and the thoughts and feelings that the therapist experiences in reaction to the therapeutic interaction. Therapists are encouraged to treat all thoughts and feelings as potentially important sources of information about the interaction with their patients. Countertransference refers to all the reactions the therapist has in the interaction with the patient, reactions that may or may not be the result of projective identification from the patient and may or may not be processed in a manner that could be labeled empathic. This definition requires therapists to contain and tolerate in consciousness their thoughts, feelings, and impulses having to do with themselves, their patients, and the dynamic interaction between them.

Working with fertility patients can arouse many countertransferential feelings in a therapist because of the intense nature of the fertility treatment process and the feelings of desperation, regret, anxiety, depression, fear, failure, guilt, and shame that are often experienced by patients. The therapist's degree of conscious awareness of her countertransference often depends on her capacity to tolerate and become aware of these powerful feelings which are aroused by the interactional communication from the patient. For example, a therapist may suppress and deny powerful feelings of hopelessness, inadequacy, and failure elicited in the therapeutic encounter because of her inability to tolerate such feelings.

Working with countertransference also involves an exploration and awareness of the therapist's own personality makeup, including ongoing conflicts and concerns that could disrupt the therapeutic process. Tansey and Burke (1989) note that this lack of awareness may result in such phenomena as enduring blind spots, rigidity, hypersensitivity or insensitivity to certain issues, and prejudicial stereotyping. Identifying global prejudices as well as specific personal biases is particularly important when treating fertility patients. Treating single mothers by choice often taps into many generalized stereotypes that may also be reflected in personal biases. It is important for therapists to know how they feel about these issues.

Some therapists are flexible and accept differences among people and may feel comfortable with a family structure that is atypical. On the other hand, some therapists might have definite ideas about right and wrong and may not be comfortable with choosing an "unconventional" path. Therapists who believe that there is only one right way to do things might have a difficult time working with patients who wish to create an alternative type of family. Therapists' relationship with their own reproductive histories and decisions about family building may influence their therapeutic work with single mothers by choice. For example, those who chose not to have children may be biased either toward or away from living child free, depending on their own unresolved conflicts with their personal decisions. Therapists who have children may be prejudiced in the direction of family building "at all costs," which may affect their treatment with a single woman who wants to stop treatment and make peace with failed IVF attempts. A therapist who adopted a child as a single woman may be biased against assisted reproduction, and her bias may affect her interactions with a patient who wishes to use donor sperm.

Working with infertility patients constantly challenges me to be aware of my own beliefs and biases and the context in which I work. I realize that I must be aware of what I bring into the room as a therapist. I enter the room as a newly married woman without children who is often challenged to confront these issues by staff and patients. Staff members immersed in the world of reproductive medicine often assume that those of us who are married but do not have children must be struggling with infertility. Patients often press for information related to my marital status, desire for children, and whether or not I have tried to conceive and had difficulty. At times I am put off by my patients' questions, which force me to confront my own ticking biological clock. Their questions challenge my confidence as a new professional in the field. Their assumptions often lead to self-doubt about whether or not I can truly grasp the painful significance of their plight without having suffered through infertility myself, which, in turn, raises fears that I might one day be faced with their same crises.

Therapists also work within a larger system, whether it is a reproductive clinic or the community where they practice. From a more systemic point of view, I am aware of my countertransferential reactions to the opinions that are held and decisions that are made by many of the male dominated reproductive programs. Many staff members believe that women should think about their priorities and potentially put aside their career or educational goals and focus their energy on having children before it is too late. My own bias is that women should have control of their own bodies, which includes their right to reproduction. I believe that women today have choices beyond the traditional view of finding their fulfillment solely within the family as wives and mothers.

It cannot be ignored however, that 42% of high-achieving, high-earning women in corporate America are childless at ages 40–55 (*High-Achieving Women*, 2001) and have not "chosen" to be that way. But what about the younger single women who want to freeze their eggs so that they can pursue children at a later time and concentrate on their careers now? Since the scientific advancement of egg freezing has shown promising results, why are practices still so reluctant to accept such patients? It appears that there may be an inherent inequality in a system that has allowed men to freeze sperm for centuries without questioning their motives or ambitions and has allowed men to continue to become fathers well past the age limits for most women in reproductive programs.

CASE EXAMPLES

The following examples have been compiled from the experiences of several therapists working in the field of reproductive medicine and have been modified to protect confidentiality. They are careful reconstructions of actual therapy cases and the therapists' reactions to their clients throughout treatment.

Anonymous Donation Case Example

Some women think they have until their 40s to decide about motherhood because of all the medical technology available today. Thus they postpone thinking about motherhood, only to realize at 42 or 43 that they are very unsure and unclear; they may also have serious fertility problems by that time. Most expect to conceive rapidly and do not realize it could take several IVF or IUI cycles before conception occurs. Most are also ignorant about the prevalence of early miscarriage or age-related genetic issues.

Helen, a 42-year-old single woman, had a secure job with a decent income. She began thinking about donor insemination several years ago and attended some Single Mothers by Choice support group meetings but could not bring herself to take the next step. It became clear that this was a type of midlife crisis for her. She was beginning the second half of her life, and she felt that in the first half she had been too devoted to meeting the needs of others. Now she wanted to do something major for herself. She had been involved in several relationships with men who were not interested in committing to anything beyond casual dating. She entertained the idea of asking one of the men she had been seeing if he was interested in donating but decided that it was immoral to have sex with a man just to become pregnant without a longer and more enduring relationship.

Helen eventually chose an anonymous donor with physical features very similar to her own and was prepared to do an IVF cycle at a reproductive clinic. Each time she came in for her blood work, she had elevated FSH levels and was told she could not begin an IVF cycle but could do inseminations. Each time she prepared for the insemination, she had an acute anxiety attack and cancelled the cycles. After her third cancelled cycle, a nurse in the practice referred Helen for therapy.

Helen came to treatment acutely anxious and noted that she had "full-blown" panic attacks that worsened the week leading up to the insemination. Helen emphatically disagreed with the therapist when she suggested the possibility that Helen was ambivalent about moving forward. Instead, Helen described herself as a procrastinator who became anxious before making big decisions. She was traditional by nature and had difficulty reconciling her choice to use a donor to have a child. She was concerned about how she would explain this choice to her colleagues, friends, and, most of all, the child.

She had grown up with an emotionally abusive father and a symbiotic relationship with her mother. One of her sisters had severe mental handicaps, and her older sister was competitive and also trying to get pregnant. Helen had discussed her plans for donor insemination with her mother, who was sometimes supportive and sometimes ambivalent and even critical. Her mother would often make comments alluding to the fact that Helen should focus her energy on finding a husband. Helen had difficulty discussing her feelings about not having found a partner and often stated that she had "given up." She was later able to understand that her failed relationships were due to her complicated and destructive relationship with her father.

She was most concerned with having a healthy child and was preoccupied with what would happen to the child if she died. She worried about pregnancy and how it might exacerbate some of her health problems. She also felt burdened with knowing that she would be responsible for caring for her mother and mentally challenged sister should something happen to either of them. She had a very weak support system and was not particularly motivated to meet people. As the therapist came to know this woman better, she seemed to be hoping for a child to love her and make her feel less lonely. She fantasized about a little girl who would love her unconditionally and take care of her when she got older. Someone who would take her away from her enmeshed relationship with her own mother, someone who would help her create a life of her own.

Helen was able to go through several insemination cycles without anxiety but became increasingly more depressed with each failed attempt. She ruminated with regret that she had not started the process years ago and was convinced that if she had tried earlier, it would have worked. She often told stories of others who had successful pregnancies late into their 40s. She rejected any comments from the therapist related to the statistics for someone her age or that she might have encountered these same problems even if she had tried years ago. Any mention of mourning the losses that she was feeling grounded her firmer in her position that this was going to work if she kept at it.

She was able to use supportive therapy to gain more insight into her motivations, to feel less depressed, to improve self-esteem, and to take more control of her life. While she was resistant to focusing on any aspect of her life that would shift her focus away from fertility treatment, she was able to understand the importance of building a stronger support system even if only to help her with the potential child. She was reluctant to explore family-building options such as adoption and donor egg/embryo. She had given up all hope of meeting someone at her age who would want children.

In the beginning of treatment, the therapist experienced many of the same emotions that Helen was feeling. She felt anxious about the level of ambivalence that Helen was experiencing and felt pressured to help her make a decision about whether or not to move forward with insemination. The therapist used these feelings to identify with Helen's present state of mind, to help her cope with her anxiety, and to explore her fears related to moving forward with donor insemination. The therapist contained Helen's confusing thoughts and feelings without the judgment, rejection or doubt that she was used to receiving from her family.

This containment allowed her the space to understand her underlying motivations for wanting a child. The therapist was initially concerned about Helen's reasons for wanting a child and was able to acknowledge to herself that her concern signified a double standard. She realized that she was more concerned with Helen's line of reasoning than she was with that of the married couples that she treated. She found herself more critical of Helen's reasons for wanting a child, even though these same reasons had been expressed by women with partners seeking insemination. She understood her bias and her view that in a two-parent family the child has double the probability that one of the parents will be a natural fit with the child. The therapist was concerned that, since Helen was the only one providing security and nurturing, she would have to work harder to find a way to adapt to the child. The therapist was feeling overwhelmed with many of the fears that Helen was reluctant to talk about and used these strong concerns to help Helen think about how she would feel if the child's temperament, health, gender, looks, and personality did not come close to the baby of her dreams.

Helen remained hopeful during the first few cycles, but her reaction to the failed attempts began to change and take on a more obsessive quality. In the subsequent sessions, Helen began to focus on the reasons why the treatment had failed and what she could do differently the next time. She quickly shifted from discussing the motivations for wanting a child to concentrating on the next scheduled cycle and medical protocol. As the treatment unfolded over several months, the therapist's countertransference response to Helen also changed.

The therapist became aware that her initial positive regard for Helen and shared hope for a successful outcome had shifted to genuine concern about what would happen if the cycles were actually successful and Helen became pregnant. Aware of this gradual shift, the therapist decided to work directly with her feelings within the session. When she commented on her observations that the two of them had been so focused on discussing the "failed" cycles that they had not talked about what would happen if Helen achieved a pregnancy, Helen became tearful. She admitted that she had been working so hard toward achieving a goal that she had lost sight of and completely avoided the outcome. She had come to expect "failure," which had allowed her to continue cycling without anxiety or fear. Her only concern was that her physician would tell her that she could not try again. She spent a few sessions revisiting her fears about "success" but gradually became resistant to any of the therapist's interpretations related to the reality and probability of a pregnancy and delivery given Helen's diagnosis and age.

The therapist felt frustrated with Helen's level of denial and was concerned about her determination to continue treatment indefinitely. Helen began to cancel her therapy appointments and the therapist began to feel rejected and wondered if she was "too hard" on Helen. The therapist's attempts to get the patient to come in and talk failed, and the therapist gradually became part of the larger system that Helen desperately feared would ultimately reject her and deny her the treatment that would bring her closer to fulfilling her dream of having a child.

Directed Donor Case Example #1

Mary, a successful physician, age 49, was divorced 10 years ago and had had no luck finding "Mr. Right." She had looked for someone to settle down with but found that most of the men in her age range who were interested in getting married and having a family had already done so. She was the only child of parents in their 70s and was concerned that they would rely on her more as they continued to age. On the other hand, she felt that she wanted to have a baby and be a mother before it was too late. Mary felt confident that she had the capacity to be a good parent and knew that she could afford to support a child. Her family and friends were people she knew she could depend on for emotional support.

After thinking about it for several months, Mary realized that conceiving with sperm from an unknown donor was not the right choice for her. She felt that she had to know the biological father of her child and decided to ask a long-term friend with whom she had been romantically involved in the past. She described this man as her best friend. Though she occasionally had had sexual relations with him, she noted that he had been living with another woman for several years.

Mary indicated that she preferred to have a child with him "naturally" even though he told her that he did not want to have a child through sexual intercourse. He had not told his current girlfriend about his plans to donate sperm to Mary. It appeared that Mary and this man had discussed the financial, emotional, and legal boundaries of their directed donor arrangement and felt comfortable with the process. He planned to be an active part in the child's life but did not plan to disclose that he was the child's biological father. Mary seemed to go along with his wishes although, at times, she indicated frustration that the relationship had remained platonic and that she would not be able to disclose fully the arrangement to the child.

When questioned about potential future complications with this man and his relationship with her and their child, she acknowledged that it might be complicated but she was determined to move forward. She told her reproductive endocrinologist that the couple were married for fear that he would not treat her if she were a single woman with a known donor. She seemed unconcerned that the sperm would not be quarantined because of the clinic's assumption that they were married.

She attempted several unsuccessful IUI cycles and noted that she was feeling increasingly powerless with each failed attempt. After a few sessions, she stopped therapy but called several months later in crisis. She was about to start medication for an IVF cycle using the same donor but had since become involved in a relationship with a man who wished to use his own sperm. She was conflicted about how to tell the donor and feared that the program would not allow her to switch donors especially since they were under the impression that she was already married. She was encouraged to discuss with her physician the possibility of delaying treatment so that she could come in for counseling both alone and with her new boyfriend.

It is sometimes difficult for a therapist to separate her own views of the situation from the patient's views. This awareness is important so the therapist can shift from what she might do in any given situation to what the patient might do in the situation. Doing this requires a constant check of her own countertransference so that the therapist may assume the subjective perspective of the patient while paying attention to her own experience of the interaction at any given moment.

This case stimulated many complicated feelings for the therapist. What do you do when you think a runaway train is heading for a tragic crash and your patient doesn't even realize that she has boarded the train? Is it the therapist's job to steer the train onto another track when it is the clear wish of the patient to keep it moving ahead full force?

The therapist felt challenged to balance her gut feeling that the situation (with the original donor) was a disaster waiting to happen with what she considered her nonjudgmental role as a therapist. While she tried not to let her feelings get in the way of treatment, she attempted to find ways to use her reactions to serve what she thought was the best interest of the patient and the potential child. The therapist openly expressed many of her concerns about Mary's initial choice of a donor. She worried about Mary's fantasy that the donor would leave the woman he was dating for Mary once the child was born. The therapist felt that she was colluding with Mary and her donor in supporting the donor's infidelity. She was worried about Mary's last-minute switch of donors and her resistance to thinking through all the issues. She encouraged the patient to be forthcoming with the program regarding the fact that she was not married. She was uncomfortable with Mary's lying to the practice but felt that her hands were tied because of confidentiality.

She knew that Mary was determined to move forward with her plans regardless of what anyone told her. Although the therapist hardly ever agreed with Mary's choices, she felt that expressing criticism would only drive the patient further away from opening up and exploring the issues. She felt strongly that abandoning Mary during this life crisis would do far more harm than tolerating her own discomfort and providing a safe place for Mary to discuss her feelings. The therapist continued to voice her concerns and point out the red flags but, ultimately, had to be comfortable knowing that this decision was not hers to make.

The therapist was also aware of her own prejudices and how they affected this case. She was biased toward using anonymous donation because she felt that the boundaries were clearer and better defined for all parties involved. The therapist was concerned about the original donor's desire to be a part of the child's life without disclosing his genetic connection. Even if the parents were in agreement, she feared for the psychological health of the potential child and what his or her desires and questions about this man might be in the future. Her concerns raised many questions about disclosure. What should the child be told about the father? How could the child be protected from others asking about the father?

The therapist was also cognizant of what she brought into the room as a married woman who had experienced pregnancy, childbirth, and motherhood. She questioned how her patient would deal with the emotional stresses in raising her child alone and worried that Mary was not being realistic about the donor's involvement. She wondered if Mary's recent involvement with a new man was her attempt at acknowledging her own doubts and confirming her deeper desire to parent with a partner who would be attentive and provide support.

Directed Donor Case Example #2

At midlife, between a third and half of all high-achieving women in America do not have children. By and large, these high-achieving women have not chosen to be childless. The vast majority yearn for children. After age 40, only 3%–5% of those who use assisted reproductive technology actually succeed in having a child. Sarah is a corporate executive who realized at 43 that she was at the point where it was now or never to have a baby. Sarah is an only child of holocaust survivors and very much wanted to have a family to remain connected to her ancestral ties. She always wanted children and thought that she had plenty of time until she was diagnosed with premature ovarian failure. She was conflicted between wanting to find a partner to settle down with and wanting to have a child before it was "too late." She understood that choosing to go down the reproductive path as a single woman could potentially hamper her ability to find a partner, and she did not want to give up either option. Feeling stuck, Sarah initiated therapy to explore her thoughts and feelings about having a child as a single woman.

She decided that she did not like the idea of anonymous sperm donation and was able to find a handsome, successful, Ivy League graduate who she thought would make an ideal donor. He agreed to donate his sperm, the appropriate legal documents were signed, and four vials were frozen and quarantined for six months. During those six months, Sarah and the donor became closer and started to date. She began to have a sexual relationship with this man and hoped that she would get pregnant on her own without the help of assisted reproduction. After several months the relationship ended.

At that point, he told Sarah that he did not want her to use his frozen sperm, but Sarah, being legally entitled to the sperm, felt otherwise. Even after several sessions spent discussing the potential problems of using his sperm and the advantages of choosing an anonymous donor, Sarah went forward with IVF using the frozen sperm. She was convinced that, when the child was born, "the donor would not be able to resist" and would naturally want to be a part of his child's life and, by extension, part of her life.

Four good-quality embryos were transferred, and she was sure that the transfer would result in a positive pregnancy. Sarah was devastated when she received negative results. She became depressed, began taking Prozac, and decided to take a break before she attempted another cycle with the remaining frozen sperm.

During her break from reproductive treatment, Sarah decided to concentrate once again on finding a partner and began internet dating. She met someone that she felt a "real connection" with but did not tell him about her previous IVF cycle or issues with reproduction for fear that he would be "scared away." Feeling that her window of opportunity to have a child was closing, she attempted another IVF cycle with the remaining frozen sperm. At the point when the embryos were going to be transferred, she felt conflicted and decided that she had to tell the truth to the man she had been dating. This conflict resulted in a crisis in the relationship that led to her decision to freeze the embryos prior to transfer. Her partner, who did not know much about reproductive medicine, assumed that this meant the embryos no longer existed. Sarah wanted to do another IVF cycle using her partner's sperm, but he did not feel ready to pursue this option. They came in for counseling together, and her partner shared that he was a traditional man who wanted to be married first before having a child. It was evident that he did not fully appreciate the idea of Sarah's ticking biological clock, nor did he realize that she had frozen embryos with donor sperm that she could use at any time. He was confident that they would be able to get pregnant the "old fashion way" and responded to the reproductive endocrinologist's warnings by stating, "They are just statistics."

Sarah planned to move forward as quickly as possible with the marriage and felt confident that she would be able to convince her partner to try an IVF cycle. She continued to monitor her hormone levels, which indicated with increasing probability that she could not get pregnant using her own eggs. To complicate matters further, her reproductive endocrinologist recommended, on the basis of hormone test results that indicated advancing reproductive age, that she consider egg donation. Sarah was torn between going through with the marriage and moving forward with donor egg so that she could preserve her husband's genetic continuity or using the frozen embryos that would allow her to pass on her own genetic code. She even considered using donor egg and donor sperm if her boyfriend did not cooperate with her requests and if the frozen cycle were unsuccessful.

This case brought up several countertransference issues for the therapist. The therapist was aware that she scrutinized single women seeking assisted reproduction more carefully than she did their married counterparts. She also realized that she was questioning her patient's motives to get married more than she had with couples who stated that they were recently married because they had decided to start a family. She somehow felt responsible for the decisions that were about to unfold and worried that, like so many other infertility patients, this patient's desperation and goal-oriented mindset might be clouding her ability to make sound decisions. The therapist felt that, on one hand, Sarah might live with regret the rest of her life if she did not move forward with some form of assisted reproductive treatment; on the other hand, she felt that Sarah was pushing forward with marriage for the "wrong reasons," especially when there were other ways to have a child.

The therapist was alarmed at her own reactions when she realized that she secretly hoped that her patient would not get pregnant. She spent time deconstructing how much of her reaction was based on her patient's circumstances, and her own genuine concern for the best interest of all of the parties involved, versus the personal issues that she brought into the therapeutic relationship. The therapist had experienced her own infertility and had attempted several IVF cycles before adopting two children. Although she felt comfortable with women independently seeking donor eggs and men using donor sperm, she was extremely uncomfortable with the idea of someone creating a child using both a donor egg and donor sperm. In the latter circumstance, when neither person would have the benefit of preserving the genetic tie, she felt strongly that he or she should consider adoption.

Like the patient, the therapist was also taking care of elderly parents and felt comforted that she had adopted her own children when she was young enough that they could enjoy growing up with grandparents. She was also grateful that her children were on their own now, and she could not imagine what it would be like to be caring for a newborn at the same time as taking care of her ailing parents. Nonetheless, the therapist continues to work with this patient. The therapist's ability to explore her countertransference has allowed her to separate her own biases from her patient's desires and has helped her put aside her prejudices so that she can encourage the patient to work toward her own conclusions about her life decisions.

Therapist as Evaluator/Gatekeeper Case Example #1

Many psychologists either consult or work directly on the staff at a reproductive medicine program. Their responsibilities as psychologists on multidisciplinary teams often collide with their roles as psychologists treating patients, who expect confidentiality within a privileged relationship. This quandary brings up the issue of the therapist in the role of gatekeeper or evaluator.

In one study, the authors were very clear about their belief that single women should, on the whole, be evaluated prior to treatment (Baetens et al., 1995). They believed that choosing to become a single parent was very different from choosing to become a parent with another person. They felt that the financial challenges, the social isolation, and the kinds of reasons given for making this choice were more often problematic with single women. These authors stressed the importance of looking at the applicant's psychosexual development, childhood, family of origin, and possible early traumatic experience. They evaluated the social environment of the mothers in their study and their reasons for wanting a child. They questioned them about their disclosure stance—how they planned to explain their method of conception to their children. The primary reasons for not accepting patients were a lack of autonomy, ongoing problems with relationships, current financial or psychiatric instability or legal uncertainties, and available social supports.

Other investigators feel that single women should not be required to articulate their desire for children more clearly than married women, especially since the evidence suggests that most women have been thoughtful and deliberate in deciding to conceive (Mechaneck et al., 1988; Frank and Brackley, 1989; Leiblum et al.,

1995). Many therapists feel that single women should not be put through an evaluation of motives or psychosocial and financial status any more than married couples should and that this should be a process of discovery within a therapeutic framework rather than a test during an initial visit.

Rosenthal (1990) recommends that the counselor discuss issues of confidentiality and ask whether or not the patient wants her thoughts shared with the gynecologist. She believes that the counselor should not be the gatekeeper and noted that sometimes this role becomes cloudy and requires clarification. Occasionally, however, a physician will refer a woman for psychological evaluation for fear that she is not psychologically fit to become a parent or for fear that she may be making a hasty decision. The following two cases describe incidents when a woman may need to be encouraged to take more time and seek counseling and the support of others before proceeding with treatment.

Her reproductive endocrinologist referred Betty, a 34-year-old recently widowed woman for therapy. She had been married to her husband for five years and had conceived a child without assisted reproductive technology two years earlier but miscarried at eight weeks. The couple had difficulty trying to conceive on their own after the miscarriage and sought help with a reproductive endocrinologist and urologist. It was discovered that Betty's husband had a low sperm count, and the couple were scheduled for an IVF cycle. The husband was scheduled for a testicular biopsy to retrieve sperm. They had been advised to have back-up donor sperm available, and they were in the process of choosing an anonymous donor. Betty noted that her husband was having a difficult time accepting the idea of donor sperm and did not want to be a part of the donor-selection process. Three months before their scheduled IVF cycle, a drunk driver killed Betty's husband in a motorcycle accident. Her friends advised her to have her husband's sperm retrieved and helped her find professionals who were willing to perform this procedure posthumously.

When Betty began therapy, she was eager to move forward with IVF using her recently deceased husband's frozen sperm. She noted that she was not willing to use donor sperm as back-up and was realistic about her low chances of success with her husband's frozen sperm. Betty was advised to continue therapy and wait one year before moving forward—to allow time for grieving. Although she was disappointed, she agreed and continued in therapy once a week. She continued to go through the many stages of grieving and discussed her motivation for wanting to pursue IVF with her husband's sperm. She indicated that "This was the direction we were already going" and stated, "I want a piece of him to live on." She was close to her in-laws and felt strongly that, if she did not produce a grandchild, she would be letting them down. She even stated that she would consider using donor sperm but would tell everyone that it was her husband's child. She noted that she would never be able to forgive herself if she did not attempt to produce a child with her husband's sperm.

Certain states have attempted to pass legislation preventing posthumous reproduction, but most states have not passed laws specifically prohibiting the procedure. Consequently, as long as the state in which the procedure is being performed has not passed a law against retrieving sperm without consent, one is legally permitted to extract sperm from a deceased person and use it to impregnate his living wife. However, the American Society of Reproductive Medicine's opinion on posthumous reproduction states the following: "A spouse's request that sperm or ova be obtained terminally or soon after death without the prior consent or known wishes of the deceased spouse need not be honored." Without prior consent of the deceased person, many ethical dilemmas arise that cannot be easily resolved.

The preceding case allows for presumption of paternal permission since the couple was already planning to participate in assisted reproduction. However, the therapist felt uncomfortable having the decision-making power granted to her in this unprecedented situation. The therapist felt stuck between the program, which might decide in the end not to treat the patient, and Betty who she feared might be cooperating with treatment simply to achieve her goal of creating a child. As Betty focused on the potential insemination during each session, the therapist became more and more concerned that Betty would try to please her and show appropriate grieving so that she could "pass" and be able to move forward with her initial goal. The therapist was concerned about Betty's expectations for the success of treatment and her preoccupation with wanting to please her in-laws at the expense of what might be considered the best interest of the child. She felt protective of Betty, given her age, and the way Betty might feel when she has grieved and is in a different frame of mind.

The therapist was able to reflect on her countertransferential reactions to Betty's situation and to posthumous reproduction. She shared her concerns with Betty, and they were able to explore how Betty's current state of grieving might be affecting her motivations and decisions. They discussed the success rates of the procedure and how Betty might feel if it did not work. They explored what Betty planned to tell the potential child. Understandably, Betty was unable to think about what it might be like to date someone else in the future and how she might feel if she had a child with her husband's sperm in those circumstances. She was not ready to grasp how difficult it could be on a practical, financial, and emotional level to raise a child during grief. Betty was also unable to consider the impact of a child on her time and ability to develop new relationships in the future.

Therapist as Evaluator/Gatekeeper Case Example #2

Julia, recently diagnosed with uterine cancer, was scheduled to go through an IVF cycle and freeze embryos prior to chemotherapy and radiation treatment, which could affect her future fertility. She was referred to a therapist when she informed the nurse the day before starting the cycle that she was going to use her boyfriend's sperm rather than the previously agreed upon donor sperm that she had selected. The therapist agreed to see her that day and changed her schedule to accommodate her. The therapist made it clear that the program was concerned about her last-minute change of heart and that she had been referred to a therapist as part of an evaluation that would then be discussed with the treatment team.

Julia's medical chart indicated that she was 42 years old, but she explained that she was really 39 years old and that her parents had changed her age when she was younger so that she could skip grades in school. When questioned about her reasons for wanting to switch sperm donors, she said that her boyfriend had offered at the last minute and that he did not want her to use donor sperm. She had been dating her boyfriend for a year but had never mentioned him to anyone on the staff and had stated she was single during her initial consultation with the physician. When asked if the program could contact her boyfriend to discuss his feelings about "donating" his sperm (a routine policy at the program), she said that he was out of the country and was not reachable. She noted that if it were a problem for the program, she would do the first cycle with the donor and the second cycle with her boyfriend. When asked to explore her feelings about having frozen embryos with two different genetic sources, she seemed unaffected and stated, "I might not even use them." On further discussion, the therapist learned that her boyfriend was unaware of her cancer diagnosis and thought that she was freezing embryos as a way to safeguard her future fertility so that she could continue to pursue her career.

When she was told that the program could not move forward without her boyfriend's informed consent, she became argumentative and thought that the therapist's stance was punitive. She felt that the therapist had invaded her privacy and her right to choose what she wanted to disclose within the confines of her private relationship. Julia was very emotional during the consultation and began to decompensate. She went into great detail about other areas in her life that were "falling apart" and described a recent work "misunderstanding" that had led to her being fired. She was informed that the therapist planned to recommend to the medical staff that she postpone the treatment she was to begin the following morning. It was suggested that she talk to a therapist in greater detail about her decision to choose a known versus an anonymous donor. By delaying the process, the program could also meet with the boyfriend and the couple to determine his willingness to participate if she chose to proceed with his sperm.

Julia became enraged and began bargaining with the therapist. She begged her not to disclose to anyone the information they had discussed and suggested that they forget about their conversation. She said she would revert to the original plan of using donor sperm. She was manipulative and told the therapist that the therapist was taking away her last chance of conceiving on the basis of her age and her upcoming cancer treatment. She appealed to her physician. She claimed, "The therapist misunderstood what I was saying" and made specific demands to be evaluated by a psychiatrist outside the clinic.

After an hour and a half with the patient, the therapist felt exasperated and emotionally exhausted, which she had not felt prior to the session with Julia. The therapist had many practical concerns about allowing Julia to move forward and she felt pressured to make a decision because Julia was to begin taking IVF medication the following morning. She was apprehensive about Julia's unwillingness to be forthcoming with information about her boyfriend. She felt that Julia was lying to her boyfriend and possibly to the program, and she worried that Julia wanted the program to create embryos without informed consent from the boyfriend. The therapist was concerned about Julia's decision-making abilities and psychological stability, especially during this time of medical crises and emotional distress. Julia did not seem to realize that she could be creating potential life and appeared detached from the process. She seemed more preoccupied with her own schedule and being able to fit in two cycles prior to her cancer treatment than with the relevant psychological issues that warranted more exploration.

On one hand, the therapist felt irritated, angry, and manipulated, and, on the other hand, she felt guilty that she could be taking away Julia's only chance to have a genetically related child. The therapist was unaware of her countertransference reaction during the evaluation. Had she been able to ponder her intense reactions to the interaction during the session, she might have responded differently. The therapist wondered if Julia interacted with others in the same sadomasochistic manner alluded to when she described her recent interactions at her job. During the session, the therapist felt bullied and was trying to avoid the pitfalls of masochistic submission, at one extreme, versus sadistic retaliation at the other. It is possible that the therapist's attempt to stand up for herself and the program without becoming harsh or punitive may have been therapeutic as it is likely that she was also standing up for something in Julia, since the patient had undoubtedly been on the receiving end of what she was directing toward the therapist during the session.

If the therapist were treating this patient in therapy, she might have tried to understand in a more comprehensive way what was taking place within the interaction with Julia by using several sources of emotional knowledge about the patient. She could have drawn on her understanding of her own experience, Julia's experience, and the interactional communication between the two in an effort to give back this understanding to the patient. Depending on the relationship, the therapist might have said, "I think you are very afraid about what is happening and feel overwhelmed and may be trying to pick a fight to avoid dealing with the reality of the situation." The therapist's attempts to illuminate Julia's underlying experience of being overwhelmed with fear and concern, as well as the manner in which she was struggling to cope with this experience, both from an intrapsychic and an interpersonal point of view might have facilitated a deeper level of insight and might have forged a different patient–therapist relationship. Given the limitations of the consultation, however, these issues were never explored, and Julia was able to "convince" the outside psychiatrist and her physician that she was "fit" to move forward with the anonymous donor.

CONCLUSION

Women in need of donor sperm have come a long way since the first donor insemination when the patient was not even aware that she was being inseminated with donor sperm. Women's rights and women's diverse roles in society have shifted dramatically over the years. More women than ever before are in the work force today, and the gap between the earnings of men and of women is narrowing. This new-found independence combined with the increase in divorce rates, have left women feeling less pressure to marry. Whereas, at one time, the romantic ideal of marriage was for women to have their needs met by someone offering everything they could not possess on their own, including motherhood, now more and more women are choosing to remain single because marriage is no longer viewed necessarily as a benefit.

Today the social taboos that have discouraged out-of-wedlock births have waned, and women can achieve female adult status and motherhood outside of marriage. According to Engber and Klungness (1995), the message is becoming clear. No longer can single motherhood be explained away by phrases like urban dilemma, welfare dependency, and the demise of the family. The new single mother is shattering all previously held myths and stereotypes, regardless of how she acquired her status. Feminist Gloria Steinem stated (www.itus.org/and baby-makestwo/issue/html):

> It isn't a big number of women who are choosing to have children on their own. . . . it's just that [the] lack of shame and positive choice is new. . . . It would be okay if those women had been cast aside. . . . if they had been left, if they had been widowed, if they had been divorced. . . . It's okay for women to be victims. It's not okay for us to affirmatively choose what we want to do.

United States Census Bureau officials have acknowledged that "the tremendous increase in the number of single parents has been one of the most profound changes in family composition to have occurred during the past quarter century" (Engber and Klungness, 1995, p. 10). It is clear that there no longer is only one type of family. In fact, it is questionable whether or not there ever really was only one type of family. The nuclear family represented such an ideal that few people defined their environment as family if it did not fit the model of a stay-at-home mom, breadwinning dad, and two or more kids. But today there are families consisting of children being raised by single women, men, grandparents, gay men, lesbians, stepparents, interracial couples, and adoptive parents and in communal arrangements (Engber and Klungness, 1995).

These new freedoms, choices, and family constellations continue to challenge mental health professionals working in the field of reproductive medicine. When working with women pursuing motherhood without a partner, it is important to help them explore certain issues. Women may want to ask themselves: Why do I want a child? How might my life be changed as a single mother having a child and raising the child? What role did my parents play in my life, and will I be the same or different? What close relationships do I have for emotional support? What financial supports do I have? Why am I choosing this method of conception? What might I tell my child about his or her father and the method of conception (Rosenthal, 1990)?

It is equally important that therapists working in this field constantly check in with themselves to understand their preconceived ideas and biases that may affect their work with patients. I have grown to appreciate how important the countertransference process is in understanding what I bring into the therapy room, as well as how I may comprehend the interaction with my patients. I understand that the empathic process not only involves taking in the patient's influence, followed by analyzing and arriving at a tentative understanding of this material, but also entails the process of "giving back" to the patient. Countertransference is no longer merely understanding one's own reactions to the patient, and empathy is no longer simply viewing matters from the patient's perspective. The therapist must be objective about her own subjective experience. She must ask herself, What am I experiencing? Why am I feeling this way? How did this come about? What purposes might be served by the patient's arousing this experience within me? The interactional process represents the optimal outcome that ultimately results from answers to these questions and the successful processing of identifications that lead to emotional knowledge of the patient's experience.

REFERENCES

Baetens, P., Ponjaert-Kristoffersen, I., Devroey, P. & Van Steirteghem, A. C. (1995), Artificial insemination by donor: An alternative for single women. *Human Reproduc.*, 10:1537–1542.

Bernard, J. (1974), *The Future of Motherhood.* New York: Penguin.

Cashion, B. G. (1982), Female-headed families: Effects on children and clinical implications. *J. Marital Fam. Treatment*, 8:77–85.

Eiduson, B. T., Kornfein, M., Zimmerman, I. L. & Weisner, T. S. (1982), Comparative socialization practices in traditional and alternative families. In: *Nontraditional Families, Parenting and Child Development*, ed. M. Lamb. Hillsdale, NJ: Lawrence Erlbaum Associates, pp. 336–364.

Engber, A. & Klungness, L. (1995), *The Complete Single Mother: Reassuring Answers to Your Most Challenging Concerns.* Holbrook, MA: Adams Media.

Fidell, L. S. & Marik, J. (1989), Paternity by proxy, artificial insemination with donor sperm. In: *Gender in Transition: A New Frontier*, ed. J. Offerman-Zuckerberg. New York: Plenum Medical, p. 93.

Fox, M. (1980), Unmarried adult mothers: A study of the parenthood transition from late pregnancy to two months postpartum. *Dissert. Abstr. Internat.*, 40/09B, 4480.

Frank, D. I. & Brackley, M. H. (1989), The health experience of single women who have children through artificial donor insemination. *Clin. Nursing Spectrum*, 3: 156–160.

High-Achieving Women (2001). New York: National Parenting Association.

Jacob, M. C. (1999), Lesbian couples and single women. In: *Infertility Counseling*, ed. L. H. Burns & S. N. Covington. Pearl River, NY: Parthenon, pp. 267–281.

Kernberg, O. F. (1976), *Object Relations Theory and Clinical Psychoanalysis.* New York: Aronson.

Kornfein, M. (1985), Motherhood without marriage: A longitudinal study of elective single mothers and their children. *Dissert. Abst. Internat.*, 46/07A, 2075.

Leiblum, S. R., Palmer, M. G. & Spector, I. P. (1995), Nontraditional mothers: Single heterosexual/lesbian women and lesbian couples electing motherhood via donor insemination. *Psychosomat. Obstet. Gyn.*, 4:321–328.

Little, M. (1951), Counter-transference and the patient's response to it. *Internat. J. Psycho-Analysis*, 32:32–40.

Mattes, J. (1997), *Single Mothers By Choice: A Guidebook for Single Women Who Are Considering or Have Chosen Motherhood.* New York: Three Rivers Press.

Nadelson, C. (1978), Normal and special aspects of pregnancy: A psychological approach. In: *The Woman Patient*, ed. M. Notmant & C. Nadelson. New York: Plenum Press, pp. 73–86.

Pakizegi, B. (1990), Emerging family forms: Single mothers by choice—demographic and psychosocial variables. *J. Maternal Child Nursing*, 19:1–19.

Racker, H. (1968), *Transference and Countertransference.* New York: International Universities Press.

Rosenthal, M. (1990), Single women requesting artificial insemination by donor. In: *Psychiatric Aspects of Reproductive Technology*, ed. N. L. Stotland. Washington, DC: American Psychiatric Press, pp. 113–123.

Tansey, M. J. & Burke, W. F. (1989), *Understanding Countertransference.* Hillsdale, NJ: The Analytic Press.

Wikler, D. & Wikler, N. J. (1991), Turkey-baster babies. The demedicalization of artificial insemination. *Milbank Quart.*; 69:5–40.

Winnicott, D. W. (1949), Hate in the countertransference. *Internat. J. Psycho-Anal.*, 30:69–74.

9

MISCARRIAGE AND STILLBIRTH

Sharon N. Covington

REST YOUR HEAD

CLOSE TO MY HEART,

NEVER TO PART,

BABY OF MINE.

—Mrs. Jumbo to Dumbo, Dumbo

*I*t seems to be a truism in infertility counseling that we must walk in the shoes of our patients to understand the path they follow. While it is unknown how many therapists working in reproductive medicine have personally experienced impaired fertility, anecdotally it seems that a majority specializing in infertility counseling come to it as a result of personal experience. One survey (Covington and Marosek, 1999) found that 52% of the respondents had a history of infertility, with almost 71% having started to work in the field *after* diagnosis.

I, too, came to this work as a result of my personal experience with reproductive loss. My experience with two early stillbirths and a miscarriage between the births of my oldest and middle children occurred at a time when there were no support groups, few books, articles, or other written materials, and no standard hospital protocols for assisting parents after a perinatal loss. This was before the field of infertility counseling emerged. It was out of the depths of grief, with little from my personal or professional experience to help me understand the unique nature of this loss, that I found my path to infertility counseling.

I have worked in reproductive medicine for over 20 of the 30 years that I have been a practicing psychotherapist. I have counseled, during the perinatal and neonatal period, hundreds of parents who lost a wished-for child through miscarriage (before 20 weeks' gestation), stillbirth (intrauterine death from 20 weeks to term), neonatal death (in the first 28 days of life), or later through the termination of a pregnancy due to serious genetic or congenital conditions of the baby. I have worked with these parents in a variety of modalities, including support groups, group psychotherapy, and individual, couples, and family therapy. It has been a profound experience of witnessing trauma, anguish, and pain during a life-altering period.

Although my journey began when I was in the depths of grief, I have used this experience and the experience of my patients to continue to develop my clinical method. It is an ongoing process of intellectual, emotional, and theoretical growth. While many therapists would find the intense emotions of loss difficult to work with, I have used my experience with my patients to come to understand the power of therapy to heal the most profound loss. With my patients, I have been witness to incredible growth, change, and healing as parents grieve their losses and move forward with their family dreams. It is a great honor and privilege to work with this population, and I believe that my personal experience, despite the losses, has given me a vocation. This chapter focuses on the psychological issues surrounding perinatal loss and identifies some of the lessons I have learned as a therapist in working with these patients.

PERINATAL LOSS

Pregnancy, or perinatal, loss is a catch-all phrase for the death of a conceptus, fetus, or neonate during the continuum of conception, pregnancy, and birth (see Table 1). A *miscarriage*, or spontaneous abortion, occurs in the first 20 weeks of pregnancy and is the most common pregnancy loss, occurring in 20%–50% of all

Table 1. Pregnancy Loss Timetable

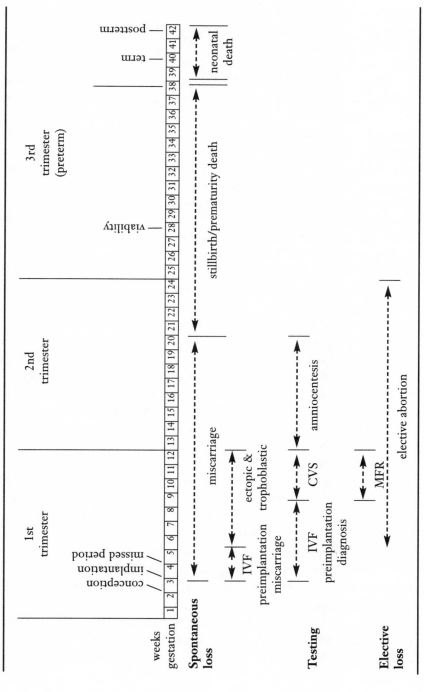

Source: Covington (1999).

conceptions. An *ectopic pregnancy* occurs in 2%–3% of pregnancies when the embryo implants and grows in the fallopian tube or anywhere outside the uterus. More rarely, *trophoblastic disease*, or molar pregnancy, happens in one out of 2000 pregnancies when the fetus dies but the placenta, the chorionic villi, or both continue to grow rapidly in a cancerlike way. Both ectopic and molar pregnancies are medical emergencies that may affect future fertility. *Stillbirth* involves the death of a fetus in utero after 20 weeks' gestation and before birth and occurs in 1–2 of every 100 births. The death of a newborn before 28 days of life is termed *neonatal death* and occurs in one out of 100 births, and may involve prematurity, birth defects, or sudden infant death syndrome (SIDS). Finally, the term elective abortion applies to the voluntary termination of a pregnancy, whether or not the fetus is viable.

Assisted reproductive technologies have further broadened the definition of pregnancy loss. For example, during IVF, conception takes place in the laboratory and, if implantation does not result after transfer of the embryo, it might be called a *preimplantation miscarriage*. Further, the development of genetic testing of fertilized eggs during IVF has resulted in *preimplantation termination* of genetically defective embryos before transfer. Finally, as a consequence of multiple gestation following IVF, *multifetal pregnancy reduction (MPR)*, or selective reduction, was developed to terminate a preselected number of fetuses in a multiple pregnancy, usually to maximize the viability of the remaining fetuses or protect the health of the mother.

Grief following a perinatal loss is acute, powerful, and all-encompassing. Intense feelings of shock, disbelief, anger, blame, rage, shame, guilt, anxiety, and depression occur unpredictably and repetitively, seemingly peaking somewhere between three and nine months following the loss (Covington, 1999). Physical manifestations of grief may include aching breasts and arms, difficulty sleeping, nightmares, lack of appetite, heart palpitations, shortness of breath, difficulty concentrating, forgetfulness, tiredness, and problems healing physically. As time passes, "shadow grief" remains, relating to a parent's desire never to forget the baby as well as the couple's general inability to express the feelings to others (Peppers and Knapp, 1980). Like a shadow, the lost baby is always there, and the memory can be triggered around significant dates and events, such as the due date, anniversary of the loss, or holidays and seasons of the years. Mourning any loss is highly individual, depending on one's personality and life experience, and will be experienced differently by each person within a relationship.

While many expressions of grief or loss are universal, there are unique aspects to perinatal bereavement that complicate the mourning process. Most significant is the *prospective* nature of perinatal grief, where mourning occurs for the hopes, wishes, and fantasies of the *future*, for a baby known in the parents' dreams. When memories of a life are primarily imagined, grief takes on a new dimension—the ineffable pain of not ever knowing. It may be a couple's first experience with death and is different from other losses in which grief is *retrospective*: that is, real memories and experiences are mourned and shared by others. Also, the narcissistic nature of the loss affects feelings of grief, mothers often experiencing intense guilt, shame, envy, rage, and self-blame.

Often there is little opportunity for emotional preparation, what I think of as "anticipatory grieving," for the loss may occur suddenly and without warning. In some situations, there may not be any visible evidence of a loss (as in early miscarriages) or an "object" to mourn. Thus it is difficult to find socially acceptable avenues to acknowledge the loss (e.g., a funeral, a ritual, or a cultural tradition) and facilitate grieving. Because the loss is invisible to many others, there is a remarkable lack of social support and parents feel it is "unspeakable," frequently being glossed over or minimized by others. Consequently, couples often find themselves suffering intense emotions in virtual isolation.

This lack of acknowledgment exacerbates a deep sense of shame and personal failure, especially for mothers. Resolving perinatal grief takes far longer than most people anticipate, from a few months to several years, and usually depends on a couple's ability to find avenues to acknowledge the loss and express their emotions. In most cases, it becomes a permanent fixture to the sufferers' psychological landscape.

Perinatal loss is a psychically traumatic event affecting how a couple sees themselves as individuals (intrapsychic), as a couple (interpersonally), and within their projections of the familial context and cultural milieu of the world around them. As in other trauma situations, parents experience flashbacks (or what I call the "psychological videotape"): intrusive and distressing thoughts and images of the event; nightmares; and avoidance of situations that trigger feelings (e.g., seeing babies). There is often an uncontrollable need and desire to replay the psychological videotape as a means of reliving and working through the traumatic experience, and this video can be recalled with precision and accuracy even years later. In fact, it is necessary for parents repeatedly to relive, remember, and discuss the experience in order to obtain distance and heal from it.

There are several risk factors that may complicate the already difficult task of mourning a perinatal loss (Covington, 1999). Generally speaking, the more intense the psychological attachment to the baby, the more significant the loss experienced by the parents: a psychological history of poor functioning, including depression or other psychiatric and personality disorders, is the single greatest risk factor for complicated bereavement.

- *Medical history* associated with the loss, including genetic issues, lupus, hypertension, cancers, gestational diabetes, Group B Streptococcus, blood disorders, and overall physical health problems;
- *Medical interventions* to achieve or maintain the pregnancy, including high-tech infertility treatment, high-risk pregnancy, extended bed rest, and selective reduction or amniocentesis prior to the loss;
- *Age*, including older women facing the biological clock and very young women lacking emotional maturity, social support, and resources to deal with the loss;
- *Marital instability*, including conflict, divisiveness, and difficulty, particularly regarding the pregnancy;
- *Social isolation*, with less emotional support and fewer resources available;
- *Other recent crises or losses*, such as another death in the family, a move, or job problems; and
- *Unrelated past trauma* and loss may be rekindled and ignited especially by something somehow suggestive of the trauma of reproductive loss.

While any of these factors may influence psychological attachment to the developing baby and intensify the grief reaction, the kind of loss—whether early or late in pregnancy—does not appear to be a determinant in grief and mourning. For example, it has been demonstrated that grief may occur after an unsuccessful IVF cycle, when conception took place in the laboratory dish but did not result in pregnancy (preimplantation miscarriage) (Greenfeld, Diamond, and DeCherney, 1988).

Grief is typically intense but begins to decline after the first year of bereavement (LaRoche et al., 1984). Pathological grief is described in terms of psychiatric symptomatology, the absence of grief, or intense grieving beyond the first year that affects the long-term functioning of the person. There is considerable evidence of disordered or pathological grief following a pregnancy loss, with possibly 20%–30% of women experiencing significant psychiatric morbidity (Zeanah, 1989).

Intervention following a perinatal loss has an impact on grief through actions that acknowledge the reality of the loss and encourage emotional expression. Supportive, reality-enforcing interventions by caregivers to parents, such as encouraging parents to see, touch and spend time with their baby, promote healthy mourning by making it real and tangible. Planning and participating in mourning rituals such as a funeral, a memorial service, a tree planting, or making a memory box help facilitate grieving. Open, compassionate communication by caregivers regarding medical information, follow-up care, and grieving, as well as referrals for support groups and counseling, have been shown to shorten bereavement (Covington, 1999).

Acceptance, or "resolution," occurs when the loss has been integrated into the patients' lives and no longer consumes all the couple's focus and energy. The couple expands their attention and emotions to include aspects of experience beyond mourning and grieving. This movement may occur when the couple has found the inner resources to move on or when life's events draw the couple out of grieving. This point may coincide with a subsequent successful birth, which appears to be an important contribution to the resolution of perinatal loss for some women (Cuisiner, Janssen, and de Grauw, 1996). For many women, another pregnancy is an opportunity to "redo" a failed experience and regain feelings of competency and accomplishment with a successful birth. This subsequent pregnancy, however, will often be shadowed by the prior traumatic loss.

While most women experience a profound "hole" in their lives following a perinatal loss, some imagine that getting pregnant quickly will make them feel better, thereby replacing the lost child and filling the hole. The pregnancy then serves as a means of avoiding grief and may affect the relationship with the subsequent child (Zeanah, 1989). However, each prospective parent needs to have sufficient opportunity to heal physically and emotionally before attempting the challenge of another pregnancy. Frequently, it is helpful for the therapist to acknowledge that this dual healing takes far longer than most realize, and getting pregnant too quickly after a loss often complicates the difficult task of grieving while dealing with a highly anxiety-producing pregnancy.

Over the years, I have taken an eclectic approach to perinatal bereavement therapy based on psychodynamic and cognitive-behavioral theory. I tend to be quite active and interactive. I advise, analyze, educate, advocate, console, and support while employing a variety of treatment modalities: individual, couples, family, support, and therapy groups. In the following case vignettes, I have identified several situations surrounding loss issues and treatment approaches, which I believe are representative of much of the work that I do.

CASE VIGNETTES

Multiple Miscarriage: Lacey and Jack

Lacey and Jack, in their late 20s, came to see me following their fourth pregnancy loss. Two years earlier, in her first pregnancy, Lacey had delivered an 18-week baby girl who died when Lacey's water broke and the baby was too premature to survive. They were living in a new city, far from their families, and had few friends. They declined to see their baby, have a memorial service, or recognize the loss in other ways, despite the hospital's suggestions. They briefly attended a perinatal loss support group but stopped when they decided to move back home. Jack's father had been recently diagnosed with lung cancer, and they wanted to be closer to family.

Lacey got pregnant several months later but had an early miscarriage. She experienced abdominal pains, and it was discovered she had multiple ovarian cysts that required abdominal surgery. With each reproductive problem, Lacey's self-image was more damaged. She subsequently had two more surgeries and miscarriages before she came into therapy depressed, anxious, and feeling her body was a "toxic waste dump." Jack, who came to the sessions to support his wife, denied any grief ("You have to be positive and just move on"), yet he was working longer hours and drinking more in the evenings "to unwind." Lacey's family minimized the miscarriages and did not seem to understand their losses. Jack's family was focused on his father, whose condition was terminal. Lacey was terrified of getting pregnant again, yet both she and Jack longed for a family and needed to cling to each other as their families of origin distanced themselves.

This case illustrates several common themes, including that each loss, building on the prior loss, magnifies the pain and makes the work harder. Lacey's self-image was shattered by the repeated miscarriages and surgery that made her feel she could not trust her body or doctors. Any ache or pain became magnified and debilitating as her fear grew. She became very focused on, even hypervigilant about, her health and often researched health issues on the internet. Any visit to the doctor could precipitate an anxiety attack. Lacey had great difficulty letting others help her. Jack needed to know that his support was necessary, and his presence was important at all medical appointments. Lacey also needed to know she could count on me, and I encouraged her to call between sessions if she was overly anxious. With Lacey's permission, I spoke with her doctor. We agreed that, rather than feeling she had to figure it out alone, she should call or set an appointment if she had any health concern. Lacey felt abandoned by her mother and needed my modeling to show her how to care for herself.

In many ways, Jack was trying to avoid grieving by letting Lacey do the emotional work for both of them; he feared the loss of his father and future family at the same time. As Lacey's anxiety diminished, Jack was able to see that work and alcohol were defenses against his sadness, and he began talking about it. The couple avoided taking concrete steps to acknowledge and recognize the losses in a tangible way. Their inertia was supported by the extended family's resistance.

To begin the emotional work together, I encouraged Lacey and Jack to find ways to acknowledge these losses as real and worthy of being grieved (see Table 2). They planned a memorial service in their backyard for just the two of them, reading poems they had written and planting a small rose garden with a bush for each baby.

As Lacey and Jack took tangible steps to work through their grief, they began the next important step in the work—future plans for a family. A fundamental reality cast a shadow over the hope for a future pregnancy: Lacey was not sure she could deal with another loss. She needed to hear from Jack that he understood and supported her. I knew that Lacey needed an "out." Encouraging them to explore adoption, I told Lacy in a somewhat paradoxical way that she did not have to go through another pregnancy to have a family. I suggested they make an appointment with their doctor to make sure they had all their medical questions answered and develop a "pregnancy plan" to monitor the next pregnancy before making a decision. I consciously tried to remain neutral about their future plans and not allow myself to be invested in either outcome. After Lacey and Jack attended an adoption seminar, their ambivalence about attempting another pregnancy diminished. After several months, they were clear that they wanted to try "one last time" and, if they had another loss, they would then pursue adoption.

Lessons Learned:

- Lacey's experience reminded me of my earlier experiences when there were no supports for my losses or tangible ways to mourn. Couples need help in taking steps that acknowledge the loss and facilitate grieving, thereby diminishing isolation.
- I created a holding environment for intense emotions induced by Lacey and Jack and served a stabilizing function. This couple needed a safe place to feel their intensity of grief, which their families and friends could not tolerate.

Table 2: Interventions after Perinatal Loss Which May Facilitate Grieving

Medical:
- ☐ Choice of induction/delivery plan
- ☐ Seeing, touching, spending time with the baby or viewing products of conception
- ☐ Naming the baby
- ☐ Taking pictures (if declined by parents, stored in record for later availability)
- ☐ Providing mementos—lock of hair, wristband, foot prints and hand prints, length/weight certificate, symbolic representations, sonograms
- ☐ Plan for disposition of body/tissue
- ☐ Funeral or memorial service
- ☐ Choice of room assignment off OB floor or discharge planning
- ☐ Providing written materials on perinatal grief and support resources
- ☐ Interim telephone call from staff before follow-up office visit

Psychological:
- ☐ Creating a memory box or album—photographs, sonogram pictures, laboratory reports, IVF petri dish, cards, toy or item of clothing, and so on
- ☐ Memorial activities—planting a tree, selecting a garden statue, donation to special charity, books for support groups, items for NICU or high-risk unit, and so on
- ☐ Self-care activities—regular exercise, proper diet, avoidance of alcohol and drugs, following a schedule/routine
- ☐ Keeping a journal, diary, or audiotape describing the loss and grief
- ☐ Writing a letter or poem of goodbye to the baby
- ☐ Planning a memorial service, private or with others
- ☐ Reaching out to a support group or family/friends

Source: Covington (1999).

- Couples need to grieve each loss before attempting another pregnancy; and, when they feel emotionally stuck it is usually because they are unconsciously resisting their grief.

Loss after Infertility Treatment: Henry and Susan

Henry requested therapy for himself after losing twin daughters at 24 weeks' gestation. His daughters had been conceived through IVF. He and Susan had been through three years of infertility treatment and were overjoyed when they learned they were expecting twins following their second IVF procedure. They were devastated when Susan prematurely delivered them owing to an incompetent cervix. Several months had passed since the funeral, and Henry had become more depressed, isolated, and withdrawn. While family and friends would frequently ask about Susan, no one ever asked Henry about his feelings. He felt he was doing "much worse" than Susan, who did not want to talk about the experience. She would say, "It doesn't help." He had no interest in resuming sexual intimacy; he felt that he had become "just a sperm donor." Susan wanted to start IVF again as she felt that being pregnant was the best way to get over her grief. Henry was unable to say no as he very much wanted a child.

This case underscores that fathers are often the "forgotten mourners" and that it is important to involve both partners in the process to support the relationship. Henry was experiencing a bit of a role reversal, as he was the "guardian of feelings" in the relationship. He was the youngest child, with four older sisters. He felt out of control with his sadness and had difficulty finding ways to express it. I found myself feeling angry with Susan and realized that I had identified with Henry's dissociated feelings. He was unconsciously angry with Susan for shutting him out during the infertility and loss of the twins. He turned the anger inward, and that caused him to feel depressed, inadequate, and impotent.

With Henry's understanding and permission, I was able to involve Susan in the sessions, by framing a phone call to her as a way of preparing for future IVF treatment. After several couple's sessions and after a level of trust had been established, Susan was able to see that her resistance to grieving was a defense against feeling consumed by sadness and that she needed to take responsibility for her feelings. I reassured her that Henry and I would be there to help her with her grief, and that it was my job to make sure that the sadness did not take over her life. As Susan became more depressed, Henry became less so and was able to help and support her.

In addition to our couple's therapy, Henry and Susan joined my short-term couples' pregnancy loss support/therapy group, which helped to normalize the grief experience and diminish isolation. During several of the sessions, my cotherapist and I divide the couples so that the men and women meet in separate groups. This technique has been particularly helpful for the men, who would not likely join a group by themselves yet long for the opportunity to share their experience with others. The men frequently share, as Henry did, feeling marginalized and ignored by their medical caregivers.

Like many infertility patients, Henry and Susan had become so focused on having a baby that their marriage suffered. The infertility had created a life of its own with repeated cycles of hope and sadness, anxiety and depression as the couple attempted pregnancy. The couple needed to step back to remember what had brought them together in the first place. I reminded them not to lose sight of their relationship in their struggle to have a family and that they needed to rediscover the things in the past that helped them feel close and intimate. Establishing sexual intimacy was essential, and I encouraged them to reclaim their sexual relationship by focusing on lovemaking and delaying "babymaking." After several months, when they were feeling much better and closer, they attempted IVF again and became pregnant. I had continued to see them through the time of their last loss, a point at which couples start to feel better and need less support. Being able to overcome the loss places them in a time when they have never had a problem and their healthy defenses are more intact. Henry and Susan had a healthy baby boy and are doing well.

As they move through their grief, I often try to help couples discover what I call "The Gifts" their lost baby has given them. In this case, it was Henry and Susan rekindling their marriage and learning communication skills that would help them throughout life. By identifying these gifts, couples are able to feel comfort knowing that their lost child lives on in their hearts.

Lessons Learned:

- Men's grief can be as great or greater than women's and should not be overlooked. Couples often "balance" their grieving; as one is more depressed, the other may be less.
- Infertility and perinatal loss together complicate grieving. Before trying again, couples need to heal their relationship, sexually and emotionally, because it has been affected by the infertility.
- During a subsequent pregnancy, passing the gestational time of loss often diminishes anxiety.

Loss Due to Baby's Defect: Sherry and Bob

Sherry and Bob were both successful, attractive professionals who had carefully planned and prepared for their first pregnancy. Sherry requested therapy shortly after delivering a 21-week still-born baby boy with a serious and rare genetic defect that causes sympathetic health complications in the mother. While my therapeutic approach is to work with the couple from the onset, Sherry wanted to come alone, as she believed she "had the problem." She had been ill for several weeks before and after the delivery owing to infection and severe water retention. She felt horrified as her body suddenly swelled by over 40 pounds in a few days, and she described her normally petite figure as being transformed into that of a sumo wrestler. Due to Sherry's serious medical problem and the baby's genetic condition, which was not compatible with life, Sherry and Bob had made the anguishing decision to induce birth. The act of terminating the pregnancy caused Sherry great guilt.

Nonetheless, Sherry and Bob (Sherry's husband of three years) took many helpful actions as a couple to facilitate their grief, such as seeing their baby, naming him Ben, planning a memorial service, putting together a memory book, and receiving great support from family and friends. Nonetheless, Sherry felt overwhelmed by the depth of her grief. She was inconsolable and wondered why she couldn't "move on." She would spend most of her session crying and could not stop thinking about her baby and all the painful consequences and ramifications of what happened. Despite her deep sadness, she was functioning well in her job and other relationships and seemed to save her profound anguish for our sessions. I felt as if I were acting as a container for her despair and as a safe haven for grief.

This case illustrates the intense cathartic outpouring of emotion that usually occurs after a traumatic loss. The circumstances of Sherry's birth experience, as well as having a genetically damaged baby, had traumatized her, and she continually played her "psychological videotape." I spent the first several sessions asking Sherry to relive the experience with me: describe the pregnancy and birth; go through the memory box and journal she was keeping; and talk about her memories of Ben. I always ask parents if they had chosen a name for their baby, and then I use it when referring to their child, rather than saying "the baby/fetus/embryo." If pictures were taken, I ask to see them and then spend time "admiring" the baby and commenting on who he or she looked like. Even when there are congenital anomalies, I ask to have parents share any pictures with me as a means of validating their baby when other family and friends may have been afraid to see the child. I believe the therapist has to be willing to engage in "knowing the baby" as the parents have. The parents feel a painful sense of failure and, to help trust to take place, I try to validate their feelings of being good parents.

Sherry talked about singing "Mrs. Dumbo's lullaby" to Ben when she was pregnant, and now she would sing it at night as a means of soothing herself and feeling connected to her baby. With time, Sherry was able to acknowledge feeling guilty about her fateful decision. She feared that she was responsible for killing Ben. I had difficulty tolerating her guilt and self-blame and found myself reassuring her before truly understanding the origin of these feelings. Ultimately, I came to understand that Sherry's shame over this decision stemmed from her religious upbringing, work ethic, and belief that "good parents are willing to die for their children." I found that my listening, rather than correcting, allowed Sherry to move from an earlier mode of organization to a strengthened sense of self and empowered competence.

Sherry needed Bob's assistance in restoring narcissistic equilibrium from the deep wound of the traumatic birth and in healing her sense of defectiveness, an important role for husbands. Sherry had to come to see and feel Bob's needs and feel her own feelings, which helped her to be loving rather than consumed with her own pain. I helped Bob see that he needed to show his love for Sherry by frequently letting her know that she was attractive and desirable. He needed to learn that she needed his support to help her body heal, including being involved as a couple in exercise, healthy eating, and gradually resuming sexual intimacy.

Bob also needed to share his feelings about the loss and seeing his wife so ill. He stoically thought he needed to protect her from these feelings. In one session, he wept over his fears about losing Sherry, fears that overshadowed his feelings of losing Ben, which helped to lessen her guilt. In many ways, Sherry felt so responsible for the loss that she became accountable for their grief. While she attempted to protect Bob from her feelings of shame, guilt, defectiveness, inadequacy, and despair, he colluded with her, and distance developed in their marriage. As the anniversary of Ben's due date approached, Sherry and Bob decided to take a vacation where they could remember Ben and begin attempting another pregnancy. On the trip, Sherry surprisingly heard her lullaby being played on the radio and took it as a message from Ben that everything would be fine. I find that "messages" like this, from the lost child, are not uncommon and often provide a spiritual context for making sense of a senseless situation. Sherry continued in therapy, had a normal pregnancy, and terminated our work as planned following the birth of a healthy baby girl.

Lessons Learned:

- Therapists must be able to tolerate a cathartic outpouring of intense emotions: shame, guilt, anger, sadness, and defectiveness.
- When one person in the relationship assumes responsibility for the grief, it is important for the therapist to understand the function of this action for the couple.
- Husbands play an important role in helping to restore self-esteem, self-worth, and narcissistic equilibrium in their wives.

Loss Owed to Mother's Medical Condition: Jill and Tom

Jill had been diagnosed with breast cancer during her first pregnancy; then her baby died. At 18 weeks' gestation, Jill discovered a lump in her breast and subsequently underwent a lumpectomy with follow-up chemotherapy. When Jill was 25 weeks pregnant and in the middle of chemotherapy, the doctors discovered that the baby had unexpectedly died in utero, a death allegedly unrelated to the chemo. She lost her baby at the same time she was losing her hair and thus felt doubly betrayed and punished. Her husband Tom was overwhelmed, concerned about his wife's health and the loss of his daughter. He felt that he had failed to protect them both. The pain and stress were magnified for both of them because Tom had recently been laid off from work and Jill was the primary breadwinner.

It was at this unbearable point that their obstetrician referred them to me. I was overcome with a deep sense of sadness and worry when I heard Jill and Tom's story. I wondered about what it would be like to help them grieve while they were facing this health crisis. Underscoring these concerns was the need to schedule our appointments around Jill's chemotherapy schedule so that she would have enough strength to come to the sessions. However, Jill made it clear at the beginning that they were requesting my help to deal with the death of their baby and not with the cancer. While I understood that Jill needed her defenses to feel enough control to get through the chemo and thus wanted to compartmentalize the losses, I found it very difficult to ignore "the elephant in the consulting room." Jill and Tom were grieving not only the loss of their daughter but also the potential for future children as a consequence of cancer treatment and prognosis. We focused more on facilitating their grief than on healing the narcissistic wounds as it was so closely tied with the cancer.

I was conscious of trying to support their strengths, being positive, offering direction and resources, while trying not to take away any of their defenses. Also, I felt very protective of them and found myself wanting to take care of them by adjusting fees and appointments and sharing information. They abruptly stopped therapy following Jill's due date, which coincided with her ending chemotherapy. She said that they were "feeling better and ready to move on." While passing these significant dates and events may spur a flight to health, I was concerned that my need to protect and care for them may have reinforced a sense of inadequacy. I do not know what happened to them and wonder today about how they are.

With the abrupt termination, I felt their loss and worried that I might have done something wrong to make the couple flee. Did they experience my flexibility as a lack of clarity and safety? Did my willingness to adjust their fee further induce feelings of shame? Jill and Tom's withdrawal from the relationship made me feel abandoned and responsible. In some ways, their loss was acted out with me, and I internalized their projections. I had hopes and wishes for their future and wanted to help them maintain and achieve their dreams. My maternal longings gave way to a sense of helplessness and loss. My hope is that my concern and caring stabilized Jill and Tom. Since they felt they could survive on their own, this couple moved on, not wanting to lift denial, repression, and dissociated feelings.

Lessons Learned:

- Therapists need to start where the patients are and not where we think they should be. This couple wanted the right to grieve the death of their baby undistracted by other crises: they wanted to deal with one loss at a time.
- Defenses serve a purpose and need to be respected, especially when one has been psychologically traumatized. Following perinatal loss, the more defensive a patient is, the more supportive the therapist must be.
- It is difficult not to know the end of the story when we deeply care about the outcome.

Unexplained Loss: Mary and Michael

Mary and Michael came to see me several weeks after delivering a full-term stillborn son, Paul. They were preoccupied with finding out why their baby had died and were angry with their doctor. Like so many, they believed that with today's technology, the doctor should have known something was wrong. Never having experienced a death in their family, they felt ill equipped to know how to deal with this loss or how to deal with family and friends. It seemed as if both their three-year-old daughter, Lexi, and their parents had regressed, with tearful outbursts, demands, and temper tantrums. Lexi had become very whiney and clingy and had started waking up in the middle of the night screaming to get into bed with them. Michael's parents were divorced, both having remarried younger partners; and complicating the situation was the fact that his father and stepmother were also expecting a baby. Mary's parents were initially supportive but, shortly after the funeral, said it was better for her to focus on Lexi and move on. Everything in the lives of Mary and Michael felt out of control, elevating anxiety for both of them.

This case shows that every couple's family history influences their ability to work through and resolve their grief. Michael's and Mary's families were unsupportive and unavailable, as they had been throughout their lives, and this crisis was no different. Michael, the oldest of three, had been the adultified child who took care of his mother and siblings after his father had left. Mary, the youngest of three children, had grown up in an alcoholic family and was overshadowed by her siblings' accomplishments. Mary and Michael had worked hard to separate and differentiate from their families and felt their marriage was successful. However, this crisis had unsettled the system and, with the couple's defenses down, the families were acting out. Much of our work focused on understanding the family dynamics and assisting Michael and Mary in setting appropriate limits and boundaries to protect themselves. I also helped them with parenting concerns, including understanding normal developmental issues with Lexi and how to help her grieve.

Mary and Michael both felt like motherless children (and childless "mothers"), and I found myself feeling very maternal towards them. They often asked me about my personal loss experience as a means of identifying with me, normalizing their feelings, and continuing their family roles of taking care of mother. Many people who are referred to me know my personal pregnancy-loss experience; 20 years ago, I cofounded a perinatal-loss support group in the Washington, DC area called MIS (Miscarriage, Infant Death, and Stillbirth). I try to process carefully these personal questions before answering and often find that it is most important to assess the meaning of my revelations rather than content.

The unknown nature of the loss, not uncommon with stillbirths, causes great anguish and anxiety. Couples often search for reasons and, when none are found, turn to folklore (e.g., "Raising your arms above your head at the end of pregnancy can kill your baby") or spirituality (e.g., "God was punishing me" or "God needed another angel") to explain the unexplainable. Or they may blame their caregivers, as Mary and Michael did, for having a false sense of reassurance that technology can keep bad things from happening. In this situation, I believed that medical negligence was not a factor but that inadequate communication was at the root of their anger. I saw one of my roles as psychoeducational, helping to educate them both medically and emotionally, so that they could make decisions about follow-up treatment and planning. I tried to direct them to appropriate medical resources to address the issues and have their questions answered. In addition, I consulted with physicians and other medical professionals to increase my understanding of the complex medical, genetic, and congenital problems associated with perinatal loss.

We spent time talking about their frustration, sadness, and feelings of helplessness (often shared by caregivers), and I suggested they write out what they wanted to say to their physician. With their permission, I called the doctor (whom I knew quite well) and talked candidly about what they needed from her. I suggested she set up an appointment at the end of the day (so not to be rushed) to go over the couple's concerns, the autopsy, and any medical follow-up indicated. Everyone felt much better after this meeting, and all were invested in working together through another pregnancy.

When Mary and Michael became pregnant again, their anxiety increased and was exacerbated by work stress, family demands, and Michael's father's having a new baby. This anxiety is common in subsequent pregnancies, and cognitive-behavioral techniques are very helpful, including breaking things into parts—that is, thinking of the pregnancy "one day at a time" rather than monthly as in previous pregnancies. Helping to contain the anxiety and sadness, I also serve as an organizing function for powerful affective states. With a baby's death at term or shortly after birth, couples never feel completely safe and talk about not letting themselves bond with the baby until they know she or he is alive and healthy. Mary needed to be reassured that her anxiety would not affect the baby and that bonding is an emotional process that was already taking place and would naturally develop without her needing intellectually to create it. Mary and Michael continued in therapy to work on family issues, strengthening their relationship, and setting limits with their families as they prepared for the birth. They were able to feel close, connected, and well grounded going into their delivery of a healthy baby girl.

They ended therapy, with my encouragement, about six months after the birth and are doing well. I felt sad to see them leave but believed they had accomplished a great deal. It was important to let them know they could continue to grow without my assistance. They send me a card each Christmas with their children's pictures and report they are all doing well.

Lessons Learned:

- A crisis like a perinatal loss can precipitate regression in any or all family members; it can recreate difficult family patterns of interaction.
- Old losses and unresolved grief from the past that may recur following a perinatal loss provides a new opportunity for growth. Couples often feel that what they learn from therapy is a gift that, like their lost child, remains in their heart.

CONCLUSION

Working with patients following a perinatal loss is both challenging and gratifying. Therapists must be able to tolerate the outpouring of intense emotion and cathartic response to mourning a wished-for child. We must be willing to engage with the couple's grief, know the baby as the parents do, and understand that healing will occur only by painfully reliving the trauma of the loss together. This requires us to be active and responsive to our patients' powerful feelings of sadness, anger, blame, guilt, and anxiety. We should help them to understand and work through these emotions as a means of resolving their grief and preparing for the future. We also need to help our patients find gifts from the depths of despair that help them put meaning to this experience. With loss comes the opportunity for profound growth and change that we, as therapists, are given the privilege to witness.

REFERENCES

Covington, S. (1999), Pregnancy loss. In: *Infertility Counseling: A Comprehensive Handbook for Clinicians*, ed. L. Burns & S. Covington. New York: Parthenon, pp. 227–245.

———— & Marosek, K. (1999), Personal infertility experience among nurses and mental health professionals working in reproductive medicine. Presented at meeting of American Society for Reproductive Medicine, September, Toronto.

Cuisiner, M., Janssen, H. & De Graauw, C. (1996), Pregnancy following miscarriage: Course of grief and some determining factors. *J. Psychosom. Obstet. Gynecol.*, 17:168–174.

Greenfeld, D. A., Diamond, M. P. & DeCherney, A. H. (1988), Grief reactions following in-vitro fertilization treatment. *J. Psychosom. Obstet. Gynecol.*, 8:169–174.

LaRoche, C., Lalinec-Michaud, M. & Engelsmann, F. (1984), Grief reactions to perinatal death. *Can. J. Psychiat.*, 29:14–19.

Peppers, L. & Knapp, R. (1980), *Motherhood and Mourning: Perinatal Loss.* New York: Praeger.

Zeanah, C. (1989), Adaptation following perinatal loss: A critical review. *J. Amer. Acad. Child Adolesc. Psychiat.*, 28:467–480.

10

WHEN THE PATIENT HAS
EXPERIENCED SEVERE TRAUMA

Robert I. Watson Jr.

---

*P*atients' reactions to trauma, both past and present, have become a growing focus of psychotherapists and psychoanalysts alike. Trauma is conceptualized in a variety of ways, but, essentially, it is the experience of being emotionally and, at times, physically overwhelmed by an event that has grave negative consequences for the traumatized person. "Psychological trauma is an affliction of the powerless. . . . Traumatic events are extraordinary, not because they occur rarely, but rather they overwhelm the ordinary human adaptation to life" (Herman, 1992, p. 33). The aftermath of traumatic events has a relatively predictable psychological effect involving changes in emotion, cognition, and memory. When one is faced with a new, but not as severe, dysregulating event, this traumatic pattern of emotional and cognitive experience may recur. This recurrence, in turn, can greatly complicate the person's reaction to the present, less severe event. When one has been traumatized, one is vulnerable to reexperiencing the psychological impact of the initial incident.

Infertility, though not as severe a trauma as a disaster or abuse, is often experienced as an emotionally traumatic event in the patient's life. It is usually unexpected and certainly has an emotionally negative impact on both the person and his or her partner. Infertility often disrupts one's general identity and view of one's sexuality (Rosen, 2002). Furthermore, if one begins assisted reproductive technologies (ART) procedures, they are themselves often experienced as traumatic because of their invasiveness. There are a host of emotional issues that result from this physical condition (Burns, 1993; Applegarth, 1996). Often one's self-concept is badly shaken. At times, patients feel shame and at other times guilt. For some, there can be an intense feeling of being betrayed by their own body. Most commonly, there is an extreme feeling of loss of control: of one's body and of one's life and expectations. One feels powerless. Often the procedures one goes through exacerbate this feeling of loss of control (Dickstein, 1990).

How patients deal with this acute loss of control is dictated by their personality style (Rosenthal, 1993). Some patients become more obsessional, needing to know more and more about their condition and possible procedures. Others, turning to a narcissistic coping style, will become concerned only with themselves, indifferent to the world and others in general (Rosen, 2002). Still others may become much more emotional, using a hysterical style to cope. It must be remembered that the behavior associated with these personality styles is the result of extreme stress and often does not reflect the usual way the patients function in the world.

While personality style has a great deal to do with how one copes with the trauma of infertility, past life events also greatly influence one's reactions. If one has had a past trauma in one's life, the impact of the present traumalike event will be multiplied and will influence one's current reaction. A variety of traumas is possible in anyone's life, and the source of the trauma can lead to very different effects on the individual. An impersonal trauma caused by a natural disaster or an accident can result in a severe but different reaction from a trauma caused by human interaction (Allen, 2001).

The focus in this chapter is on trauma caused by another and especially by actions that are malevolent. For example, early loss of a parent can be devastating and have long-term effects on any person. As a trauma, it can have psychological effects on the patient experiencing infertility since there can be variety of conflicts and deeply embedded fantasies about pregnancy and parenting. However, traumas that are the result of another's malevolent attitude toward a person can be even more devastating and affect greatly the patient's reactions to infertility and the process used to treat it. When one has been the victim of verbal or physical abuse, especially from a parental figure, the resulting reactions can be intense and overwhelming. Those earlier traumas can reemerge when new fears involving vulnerability and lack of control occur. The patient may also be subject to greater depressive reactions during the infertility experience.

An area of early trauma that is often not considered is that of early deprivation or neglect by the parents (O'Hagan, 1995). A female patient recently sought treatment because she was at the beginning stages of dealing with her infertility and found that she was becoming increasingly angry with her doctor. She left one therapist because he would not listen to her about changing a rule involving scheduling and she was having difficulty with her OB/GYN. She was currently estranged from her parents by her choice, whereas previously she had gone to great lengths to please and placate them. Her parents were very demanding of her and were extremely ambivalent about her bearing a child and, seemingly influenced by a variety of narcissistic issues, had cautioned her not to conceive. She soon revealed a history of verbal and physical abuse at the hands of a full-time nanny. While these events had an impact on her, what appears to have had even more of an effect on her was the neglect she experienced for long periods during her childhood. During her early years, from ages two to eight, she and her family lived in a castle in Switzerland. Her parents would leave her for six months each year and return to the United States since they felt it important to keep their social obligations. She often felt abandoned and terrified, having been left in the hands of her abusive nanny. While the direct abuse she experienced with her nanny was traumatic, it seems her primary reaction was to the neglect and deprivation she experienced because of the long separations from her parents.

During her struggle with infertility, the trauma of this deprivation resurfaced in the form of a great desire to bond with her specialists and for them to pay particular attention to what she felt were her needs. Dissociated aspects of this early experience of abandonment were enacted in her present relationships with these authority figures. Although there were actual events to point to in her interactions, the emotional impact of these negative interactions was primarily due to the early abandonment experienced with her parents.

She also was extremely ambivalent about her relationship with her parents. She was struggling with a desire to enlist them for aid and support in dealing with infertility but believed such an alliance could only end in disaster. She was certain they would care for their own narcissistic needs and their reputation among their friends and would not focus on her. Rather than hope and be disappointed, she decided not to be involved with them and enlisted her husband to aid her in not having any contact with them. In treatment, she had discovered that throughout her life she had felt like a narcissistic object, valued only for her appearance and social abilities. She decided to take control of her own life; not live for her parents, and regulate her contact with them—the opposite of her feelings as a child. Her parents then left for an extended stay in Asia, where her father had business. She decided to make no attempts at communication and turned to friends and a self-help group for support.

She also found that she could turn to other relatives for support without fear of rejection. She did change her infertility specialist to a doctor with a reputation for being supportive and listening to patients. As she was able to understand her emotions and her interpersonal relationships, she was able to take control and make positive changes in her life. Because of these changes, she was better equipped to go through the emotional upheaval that accompanies dealing with infertility.

While any of the aforementioned traumas can deeply affect the experience of a patient grappling with infertility, the trauma that appears to have the most devastating effect is that of sexual abuse. A victim of sexual abuse has a myriad of issues to deal with in many situations, but the issue of and the treatment of infertility is an especially difficult one.

Many of the psychological issues associated with infertility are magnified by this form of trauma. Often there is guilt, self-blame, or shame when one first becomes aware of one's infertility (Downey et al., 1989). For those who have suffered sexual abuse, infertility often is a reminder of their earlier experiences; they have these same misplaced feelings of shame and guilt, which are particularly prevalent if the abuse occurred during childhood (Herman, 1992). Patients who have been sexually abused will often look for the cause of the infertility in some action or inaction on their part and then blame themselves, feeling defective and bad.

For many patients going through infertility, the "rollercoaster" of expectations and hopes followed by sadness and loss occurring during infertility becomes a trauma in itself. Often patients expect the worst and guard against dashed hopes by having little hope. Many sexually abused patients are continually on guard against other traumas and cope by anticipating the worst in any situation. Doing so makes the long and arduous process of ART especially difficult. Mistrust is a persistent attitude for those who have been sexually abused and is especially difficult if the current situation has any sexual association.

Certainly there is an implicit cognitive and affective association between reproduction and sex. Therefore, dealing with infertility can be imbued with mistrust. It can take the form of mistrust of specific people or mistrust of the whole process. For some patients, there is also the unfortunate feeling of being treated as an object or statistic during the process. This feeling is an anathema to sexually abused patients, who have often experienced a similar attitude of callousness at the hands of their abusers.

There is, finally, the process itself that many patients find invasive and out of their control. IVF procedures are especially emotional for abuse victims since there are often feelings of loss of control and the procedures are invading the very anatomical organs that were violated during the actual abuse. All these factors make infertility, and especially ART procedures, extremely difficult to cope with for sexually abused patients without some form of psychotherapeutic intervention.

While there are many factors that affect the treatment of patients who are going through infertility and who have been sexually abused, their relational issues are often the most difficult. Early sexual abuse especially disturbs many individuals' interpersonal relatedness, and these disturbances are carried into the treatment. Many sexually abused patients have been abused by some authority figure and therefore often have negative feeling directed at authority figures. This feeling can apply to the infertility specialist with whom they consult, but it also can apply within the psychotherapeutic dyad. A myriad of transference–countertransference issues are recognized as occurring in the treatment of most sexually abused patients (Davies and Frawley, 1994). These issues are often heightened when a patient is going through the process of dealing with infertility.

Psychotherapists can be and often are caught up in the deep emotional reactions experienced by these patients. In many ways, these interactions are a primary part of the therapeutic relationship and can be a major aid in a successful treatment. To facilitate the treatment, therapists treating sexually abused infertility patients must understand and use their own emotional reactions to infertility and sexual abuse. This use of emotional reactions is often where the traction takes place in the treatment. A variety of emotional reactions and counterreactions are possible given the potent mix of emotions associated with both abuse and infertility. These reactions can be as varied as idealization of the patient to experiencing anger at the patient. For example, a therapist may find herself being more protective of the patient and wanting to shepherd the patient through the process of dealing both with infertility and with psychotherapy. One can find oneself being reassuring and making overly protective statements if one does not understand one's reactions to the abused patient who is going through infertility.

Conversely, a therapist may experience negative countertransference reactions to the patient and the process of dealing with infertility. At times, those reactions can result in the therapist's being frustrated and angry at the patient, but more often the therapist will feel angry at the process or at the infertility specialist treating the patient. Other common negative countertransference reactions take the form of hopelessness and feelings of ineffectiveness in the psychotherapy. For example, the therapist may feel that the patient will never become pregnant or that, no matter what is done in the therapy the patient will not make progress on her issues. Psychotherapists should be aware of their feelings while treating patients, especially when they are treating patients who have been sexually abused and are attempting to deal with their infertility. While it is not "wrong" to have these emotional reactions, they should be understood in the context of the patient's history and the therapist's personal reactions to sexual abuse and infertility. As Hegeman (1995) and others (Davies and Frawley,

1994) have made clear, it is in the therapeutic dyad that much of the work of change in therapy can take place, especially reviving the patient's potential for relatedness and lessening the impact of the abuse. It is also within the therapeutic dyad that issues surrounding the emotional impact of infertility can be worked through while the actual medical process attempting to deal with the infertility is occurring.

A psychotherapist hearing about abuse may experience emotions that mirror those originally experienced by the patient during the abuse, which can lead to a feeling of profound helplessness. The therapist may actually not want to formulate the experiences that he or she is going through with the patient. As Gartner (1999) has put it, "After all, trauma by definition is an event that seemed impossible in the patient's worldview, and may seem equally impossible to the therapist" (p. 257). The therapist must listen to the trauma and formulate it for himself and the patient. By listening and experiencing the patient's report of the trauma, the therapist can help the patient in their search for emotional recovery and lessen the impact of the present trauma of dealing with infertility.

It is also important that the therapist engage the patient around the present traumatic events involving the infertility itself. Experiencing infertility, especially when ART procedures are involved, is always difficult emotionally. When it rekindles old traumas, the emotions can be more difficult to experience. It is precisely then that the therapist must not turn away from his or her own emotions, but, rather, use them to help formulate the treatment. Helplessness is especially difficult, since the therapist can have little actual effect on the hoped-for pregnancy and may feel stymied and frustrated, if not helpless. These feelings can be formulated by the therapist to move the treatment forward and help demystify the experience of the patient.

Another conceptual paradigm that can aid the therapist in treating the infertile patient who has been sexually abused is that of multiple self-states and the concomitant concept of dissociation. This new look at self-organization is based on the idea that there is no unified self; instead, there are a multiplicity of self-states in all human beings (Bromberg, 1995) that have evolved out of normative dissociation (Pizer, 1996). In this theoretical conceptualization of personality, there is no unified central self, but, rather, multiple selves.

Dissociation is a process that everyone has used, first to formulate the self-state, and then to use it in everyday interactions. Patients who have been sexually abused have often developed extremely divergent self-states, which are often walled off from each other. These patients have also had to use extreme forms of dissociation to live through their abuse. A sexually abused patient can use dissociation to such an extent that the content of an experience can be completely separated from the emotion connected to it, as when the patient experiences no feelings about the actual abuse. Similarly, when a patient is in one state (e.g., "child victim"), there can be great difficulty in changing to another state, such as "competent adult." Within the relational paradigm patients can be helped not to form a unified self, but, rather, to find the capacity to cross from one self-state to another with ease. Bromberg (1996) has termed this state "standing in the spaces," meaning the capacity to be in the dissociative spaces between the self-states. A ramification of the ability to cross self-states is the ability to hold two contradictory emotional states or points of view at the same time (Rivera, 1989). When a person cannot form these links, there can be great relational difficulties.

Applying these concepts to a patient going through infertility, one can see how the trauma of discovering that one is infertile can easily challenge one's faith in oneself and the equilibrium in one's multiplicity of self-states. The patient usually has a strong concept of the "fertile self" and has little or no way of integrating the concept of the "infertile self." This can be an especially difficult process for the sexually abused patients since they have often felt unstable about their self-system and have often had to use extreme forms of dissociation. If ART is necessary, the tests and procedures can be traumatizing in themselves and may lead to further use of dissociation and building new and higher walls between self-states that then become more difficult to move between. Therefore, an aspect of treating a patient who has been sexually abused is to help lessen the pathological dissociation and help make it more possible for the patient to move between the different self-states that emerge during this difficult time.

CASE STUDY

Patricia, a 32-year-old Family Practice Fellow in a metropolitan hospital, sought psychological treatment after her second IVF attempt failed. She had taken extra time to finish both her B.A. at a prestigious small college and her M.D. She and her husband of seven years had been trying to become pregnant for two years. Both male and female factors contributed to their inability to conceive, so they were now trying IVF. They had one trial in which five embryos were transferred but no pregnancy resulted. In a second trial, the embryos were of poor quality. Patricia did become chemically pregnant for two days. She felt "great" and was "crushed" when the pregnancy did not last. She sought treatment because of the extreme stress and depression she experienced following the loss of the pregnancy. As she was moving forward with a third trial, she felt that she needed to speak about the "tangle of feelings" she was experiencing.

My first impressions were of an intelligent, somewhat driven resident who was very aware of all the medical issues involved in the IVF process. She was emotionally labile but was able to be clear and controlled in her presentation during her initial evaluation. Her childhood background was marked by great situational swings from wealth to poverty. She grew up in rural Maine, the first child of a young couple. Her father came from a wealthy Massachusetts family. Her parents divorced when Patricia was eight, and she and her siblings and mother then lived in near poverty because their father refused to support them. One vivid memory of this time was of early high school. She and her siblings were in a field digging for leftover potatoes so they could eat. At that moment, the school bus passed by, and all her friends could see her in this embarrassing situation. On the other hand, she would spend summers in Massachusetts with her father at his family home. Most important, she spent this time with her paternal grandmother, who was a self-made woman and very highly respected in her community. Patricia was close to her and found her to be a model for her own life.

Early in the treatment, she also revealed her sexual abuse to me. She had been in treatment previously and had spoken about many of the details. She first told me of her experience of rape at 17. She had been raped by a boy at a party, who wanted sex and who forced her after she said "no" repeatedly. After the incident she sought treatment and felt it had helped her deal with many of the aspects of this violation.

She also spoke about repeated sexual violations by her maternal grandmother. This sexual abuse started in early childhood and continued until Patricia was strong enough to resist it, at approximately 12 years of age. Initially unclear about these violations, she thought that she had been molested at a daycare center. It became clear that the molester had been her grandmother when she learned that there were no older women at the center and when her mother validated Patricia's memories and admitted that the same abuse had been done to her. Patricia also recalled having a passive suicidal wish at age eight. She was swimming and the tides were very strong and she remembers wanting to be pulled out to sea. This incident followed her parents' divorce and her change in financial situation. It was while her grandmother was sexually abusing her.

She was able in past treatment to overcome many of these traumas. She was a very intelligent and motivated student and was able to go to a prestigious college; she was one of the first from her rural community to go there. She took longer than usual to complete her degree, and it was there that she met her husband, with whom she was able to establish a loving and trusting relationship. She did very well academically and gained admission to medical school, where, again, she took somewhat longer than usual to complete the program. She was accepted to her residency and fellowship of choice and was doing well in her work when she entered treatment.

When Patricia first came to treatment, she was trying to decide when to have the next IVF cycle and was dealing with negative feelings toward many of her patients, who mainly had uncomplicated pregnancies. She experienced both frustration and jealousy with many of these patients, with some because the pregnancies came easily to them and with others because they would not listen to the most basic recommendations for their prenatal care. She had difficulty seeing how she could continue in her residency if she did not become pregnant. She also spoke about how the infertility had affected so many aspects of her and her marital life, ranging from her emotional reactions to the way she and her husband had sex. She spoke about how alone she felt during the infertility procedures and how frightened she felt, although she trusted her doctor. She was most affected by the extreme slide from feelings of hope and joy to feelings of despondency when she turned out not to be pregnant.

As we spoke about these issues, I recognized many of the depressive and emotional issues that one would have following sexual abuse and going through a new traumatic situation. I also felt a great deal of admiration for what she had accomplished interpersonally and academically. I especially began to feel protective of her and wanted to help her anticipate the emotional upheavals brought on by the ART procedures. After three months in treatment, she decided to start IVF again and began taking Lupron. The medication greatly affected her emotions: she would first be angry, then sad, then angry again. She felt especially out of control, which affected her sense of self, since she had been invested in self-control after her grandmother had repeatedly abused her. She particularly experienced the procedures as a loss of control and attempted to go into them as prepared as possible.

One issue that often caused her difficulty was whether she was in the patient or the professional role. It was difficult for her to be flexible in her view of herself, especially since being a patient would mean letting go of the control she experienced as a professional. She realized that she made her situation more difficult by trying to anticipate all the medical issues rather than turning them over to her doctor. At this time, I took the position that she could be a patient and let the technicians and doctors do as much for her as they would for other patients. She began to see that she could switch between the different self-states and profit from the experience.

We also began to speak about the depth of her internal distress. In the press at the time were many articles about the suppression of knowledge about sexual abuse in the Catholic Church, and she soon began to speak about her own abuse and how the present, emotionally difficult experiences in ART were reopening many of her old feelings about both the abuse at her grandmother's hands and her rape. Particularly mystifying to her at the time was the attitude of the young man who had raped her—he did not see anything wrong in what he had done. After she spoke about both abuses, I once again felt protective of her and was especially angry at the perpetrators. I was frustrated that there was nothing to do. We were able to relate many of these feelings to her experiences with infertility.

During this period of treatment, I also had feelings of frustration with my role as her therapist. I felt I could do little with the present IVF procedures and could have little effect on her present state. I did not become frustrated by the patient but, rather, felt frustrated and overwhelmed by the situation. I slowly came to see how these feelings not only applied to the issues of infertility but also were related to her past abuse. Starting with this recognition, I was able to use these feelings to understand better her present emotional dilemma and deal more effectively with my role as psychotherapist.

In the fifth month of treatment, Patricia came to a session reporting that she might be pregnant. This announcement was soon followed by her reminding me how she had been pregnant before, but it had not come to fruition. She was not going to get her hopes up only to have them dashed. It had been an especially difficult time, since she had spent the weekend with her sister and mother, who were both intensely interested in babies and spoke about little else. She did not want to tell them for fear doing so might somehow affect the pregnancy, and she was also concerned that she might not be correct.

As it turned out, she was pregnant, and she soon began to have more and more worries about the pregnancy. She often felt "sick and tired," which she thought was good, since it indicated she was still pregnant—but she also had persistent worries of losing the baby. She did begin to make hopeful plans about what she could do about her residency when she delivered in eight months. These plans were especially important because they indicated an ability to move between the concepts of self as doctor and self as pregnant woman. It soon, however, became clear she did have difficulty in moving freely from self as doctor and self as patient. In the next session, she spoke about her first sonogram; the pregnancy was going well. She also spoke about feeling foolish asking questions of her OB, questions to which she knew the answer but still needed to ask.

At this time, I was more confrontational, asking why she could not be a patient with her own doctor. It was difficult for her to move into seeing herself as a patient and to ask anything that might be interpreted as stupid. She slowly came to see that she had a right and an obligation to herself to be a patient with her doctor, move out of her rigid doctor self, and receive the reassurance and information she could get from him. Her ability to do this grew as she became more comfortable in moving between these different self-states and as she was more confident about carrying her child to term.

It was also a struggle to accept seeing herself as pregnant. This was a new way of conceptualizing her self and had the negative side of making her more vulnerable if she did lose the baby. One helpful step came when her sister offered her many of her own maternity clothes. While Patricia was ambivalent about taking this step, she accepted the clothes and felt relieved afterward. Changes in her self-concept also began to be linked with actual bodily changes. About one and a half months after accepting the maternity clothes, she became physically uncomfortable and felt that her body image had changed and began to wear them. She had put off doing this as long as possible and was finally able to accept this view of herself and her body. She also allowed herself to become more hopeful that she would actually deliver the baby.

In her seventh month, she was officially able to apply for a leave from her position. She felt that she needed to do this because of the stress she felt owing to her workload and the guilt she would have felt if something happened to the baby at this point in the pregnancy. I was pleased that she had made this decision, for I had worried about the stress of her work. Again, not wanting her to experience another trauma, I was being more protective than necessary. A week following the decision, she began to react to the change in her self-concept. She missed some of the aspects of work but primarily spoke of feeling differently about her self. She no longer thought of herself as a resident or a doctor. Who was she? She reported a dream in which she sat down near one of the medical buildings because she was tired. She was then "hassled," first by a doorman and then by the police, since she did not belong there now. Forming a new, nonprofessional sense of self was proving difficult for her, particularly because she needed to invest the pregnancy with a sense of hope in order to accept this new concept and feel that she was not simply setting herself up for a trauma she could not control. Subsequently, she was able to express much more fully and emotionally her love for the baby and her husband—quickly followed by the fear the baby might die. When a link was made between this sequence of reactions and her past traumas, she was able to see how the past events were shaping her present reactions. She was able to speak more freely about her affection and closeness to both her husband and the child she was carrying. She was also able to associate her pessimistic attitude to her mother's belief that something bad was always about to happen and one should not let one's guard down and experience joy.

In the same session, she also began to discuss her feelings of vulnerability in giving birth. She was afraid of "looking foolish" but also afraid that her rage would surface and she would hurt or verbally abuse someone. She was afraid of loss of control and injuring someone else. She was also particularly concerned about who would deliver the baby and hoped greatly it would be the doctor with whom she had worked for the last few months. She was filled with anxiety over the possibility that a "stranger" would examine her, which she readily linked to her sexual abuse. She became calmer after she had discussed this issue with her OB.

She slowly became more accepting of her pregnant self and began to allow herself to verbalize her hopes for a baby without any complications. She began to shop for the baby and started Lamaze classes. An interesting aspect of the Lamaze training was that it brought back her memories of using dissociation during the sexual abuse. She did not want to use this old defense and, in fact, wanted to stay in the present as much as possible during the birth. After only a brief exploration, I began to assure her she could be present, but I missed an opportunity to understand more fully her use of dissociation and how it affects her presently.

As her due date approached, she did become noticeably more relaxed, but some fear still remained, now focused on the possibility of having a premature child and all the difficulty it would involve. She began to be more excited by the thought of having the child and complained more about her physical discomfort. She did have one incident that was terrifying for her husband and her.

They had gone to Maine to visit her mother. She usually felt the baby move at night, and, when she felt no movement for hours, she panicked. She and her husband rushed to the local hospital. It was soon determined that there was no fetal distress. She had lived through one of the worst situations she could have experienced and, though she had been confused and distraught, she had also experienced the help and caring of her husband and the hospital staff. She subsequently became more confident that the birth would be all right.

Immediately after this incident, Patricia and her husband moved to a new apartment. They now had a separate room for the baby that she began to decorate, even allowing herself to buy a crib. She was also touched by the help her mother and stepfather gave her during the move. She was also able to discuss with both her husband and her mother the possibility of having a second child. She began to express a great desire simply to have this child and get on with her life.

She delivered a seven-pound, eight-ounce boy within a few days of her due date. She called to cancel her appointment following the birth and gave me the good news. I felt happy for her and relieved that all had gone well. The following week she came to treatment and brought in her new son. She told me about the experience and that it was not as embarrassing or as anxiety producing as she had feared. An interesting aspect of the delivery was her lack of focus on the birth itself. She reported not thinking of herself as having a baby until she saw her son's head crown. She was able to focus on the medical experience but not herself as giving birth. This was not truly dissociation but allowed her to stay in a role in which she was more comfortable. She also commented on how difficult it had been to trust her OB but reported that she had been able to do so and follow his advice and take in his support during the delivery.

After the birth, a variety of themes developed in the treatment. At the beginning, she was particularly surprised at how extremely attached she felt toward her son. She felt herself becoming close and bonded with him, and the bonding had a positive effect on her happiness. At the same time, she had to deal with her fears that something dreadful might happen to him. These fears were made worse by the vulnerability she felt as she became increasingly devoted to him. This vulnerability was heightened by the past sexual abuse and the attitudes her mother had toward danger in the world. She was able, with support and a better understanding of this emotional reaction, to reduce her anxiety and enjoy the experience more.

More recently, she has begun to bring up her feelings of frustration with him and with focusing so much of her life on parenting. She is considering return to work, but these feelings have also brought back the issues of her own incest and the fear that she might do some harm to her son. She is clear that the cycle of abuse stops with her and realizes she has the power not to lose control with him. The idea of returning to work brings up an additional conflict and worry: child care. Because she was molested by her own grandmother, it is difficult to trust someone else with her child. She realizes that she will return to work at some point and that she must learn to trust others more if she is to be able to do this without extreme anxiety and worry. It is clear that the trauma of incest will have an effect throughout her life, but she is continuing to use her demystification of the experience and her emotional growth to change her self-concept and her experience of the world.

Trauma, and especially sexual abuse, is a complicating factor for anyone going through infertility, especially ART procedures. When psychotherapy helps demystify the connections to the present traumatic events and the relational aspects of the patient grow in the therapeutic dyad, the patient can adjust to and experience the process with less anxiety and more hope. It is also possible that flexibility between self-states can be aided during this time of stress, and walls around disconnected emotions and experiences can be broken down, further aiding the patient's growth.

REFERENCES

Allen, J. G. (2001), *Traumatic Relationships and Serious Mental Disorders.* New York: Wiley.

Applegarth, L. (1996), Emotional implications. In: *Reproductive Endocrinology,* ed. E. Adashi, J. Rock & Z. Rosenwaks. Philadelphia: Lippincott-Raven, pp. 1954–1968.

Bromberg, P. M. (1995), Psychoanalysis, dissociation, and personality organization. *Psychoanal. Dial.*, 5:511–528.

———— (1996), Standing in the spaces: The multiplicity of self and the psychoanalytic relationship. *Contemp. Psychoanal.*, 32:500–535.

Burns, L. (1993), An overview of the psychology of infertility. *Infertility. & Reprod. Med. Clin. N. Amer.*, 3:433–545.

Davies, J. M. & Frawley, M. G. (1994), *Treating the Adult Survior of Childhood Sexual Abuse.* New York: Basic Books.

Dickstein, L. (1990), Effects of the new reproductive technologies on individuals and relationships. In: *Psychiatric Aspects of Reproductive Technology*, ed. N. Stotland. Washington, DC: American Psychiatric Press, pp. 123–139.

Downey, J., Yingling, S. & McKinney, J. (1989), Mood disorders, psychiatric symptoms and distress in women presenting for infertility evaluation. *Fertility & Sterility*, 52:425–432.

Gartner, R. B. (1999) *Betrayed as Boys.* New York: Guilford Press.

Hegeman, E. (1995), Transferential issues in psychoanalytic treatment of incest survivors. In: *Sexual Abuse Recalled*, ed. J. Alpert. Northvale, NJ: Aronson, pp. 185–213.

Herman, J. L. (1992), *Trauma and Recovery.* New York: Basic Books.

O'Hagan, K. P. (1995), Emotional and psychological abuse: Problems of definition. *Child Abuse & Neglect*, 19:449–461.

Pizer, S. (1996), The distributed self: Introduction to symposium on "The multiplicity of self and analytic technique." *Contemp. Psychoanal.*, 32:499–507.

Rivera, M. (1989), Linking the psychological and the social: Feminism, poststructuralism, and multiple personality. *Dissociation*, 2:24–31.

Rosen, A. (2002), Binewski's family: A primer for the psychoanalytic treatment of infertility patients. *Contemp. Psychoanal.*, 38:345–370.

Rosenthal, M. (1993), Psychiatric aspects of infertility and assisted reproductive technologies. *Infertility & Reprod. Med. Clin. N. Amer.*, 4:471–482.

11

EXTRAORDINARY CIRCUMSTANCES

Termination of Three Pregnancies Conceived with Donated Oocytes

Shelley Lee
Frederick Licciardi

*L*ittle has been published on the psychological and emotional difficulties experienced by individuals or couples who have become pregnant using donated oocytes. Marcus and Brinsden (2000) reported the termination of a triplet and a twin pregnancy in Britain after conception with donor oocyte and donor spermatozoa. Both recipients elected to terminate the entire pregnancy despite being given the option of fetal reduction. In these cases, the fact of multiple pregnancy was the reason given for termination. Neither recipient couple cited advanced maternal age or lack of a genetic link to the fetus as a factor in their decision.

Three additional cases in which the recipients of donated oocytes chose to terminate their pregnancies for nonmedical reasons are reported here. It is notable that, in contrast to the British account, these terminations involved pregnancies conceived with donor ova and the recipient husband's sperm.

These new cases were identified through a retrospective analysis of all oocyte recipients undergoing embryo transfer from January 1996 to December 2003 in a university-based fertility clinic. During this time, the clinic had 668 clinical pregnancies (gestational sac and fetal heartbeat) in the donor egg program. Personal details have been changed to protect anonymity of the clients.

CASE I

Mr. and Mrs. A, a biracial couple, presented to the Oocyte Donation Program in their early 40s. They had been married for two years, after dating for more than 10 years. Mrs. A learned she was peri-menopausal in her late 20s and was diagnosed with premature ovarian failure in her early 30s. Mr. and Mrs. A had never used birth control. The couple had no previous infertility treatment. At presentation, Mrs. A had been in menopause for six years.

Mrs. A met the reproductive endocrinologist, went through standard testing, and had surgery to remove scar tissue in her uterus in preparation for the donor cycle. The couple was interviewed and counseled by a staff psychologist prior to the oocyte donation cycle and completed psychological testing with the Minnesota Multiphasic Personality Inventory-2 (MMPI-2), a program requirement for couples using donor gametes. Neither spouse had a personal history of substance abuse or mood disorders. Nonetheless, Mrs. A's psychological testing had a mild elevation on the depression scale. A courtesy follow-up consult in our clinic was recommended but not pursued. Mr. and Mrs. A appeared to have a supportive, affectionate, and stable relationship and appeared to be comfortable with the donor option. The psychologist's report noted that they presented as "friendly, warm, caring, realistic, and practical individuals." In the interview, Mrs. A revealed that she had disclosed her intent to use donated ova to her parents and to women coworkers, all of whom had been enthusiastic about her decision. The psychologist reviewed the possibility of multiple gestation with the couple. They reported they "would be fine with twins."

The couple requested that they be matched to a donor who approximated Mrs. A's appearance. A donor was presented to the couple 11 months later, and they did not hesitate to accept her. They chose to do a shared cycle, splitting the ova retrieved with another recipient couple and thus reducing their financial costs. Prior to beginning the cycle of oocyte donation, the couple met with a nurse who reviewed the medical protocol and instructed the patient in self-administering her medications. There was no indication to the medical doctor, psychologist, or nurse that the couple had any doubts or concerns about proceeding.

Mrs. A began a cycle of oocyte donation about a year after her presentation in the clinic. She received a two-embryo blastocyst transfer and nine days later had a positive pregnancy test. Twenty-eight days after her transfer, Mrs. A experienced light bleeding and came into the clinic for a routine ultrasound. Two fetal heartbeats were identified at week 7, and at week 12 Mrs. A completed treatment in our clinic. She was referred to a high-risk obstetrician to begin prenatal care.

In her meeting with the obstetrician, a routine high-resolution ultrasound identified three fetal heartbeats. One of the embryos had split. Mrs. A was now carrying a triplet pregnancy with identical twins and a fraternal triplet.

Mr. and Mrs. A did not want a triplet pregnancy because of the high risk to the mother and the children. Working with the obstetrician, they planned for the reduction of the twins in one sack to give Mrs. A a singleton, low-risk pregnancy. At this point, Mrs. A became very depressed. She reported that she was "crying all the time" and began to doubt her desire to become a mother. Mrs. A's husband gave her the option of terminating the entire pregnancy and she chose to do so.

The infertility staff psychologist met with Mrs. A prior to the scheduled termination. In the interview, Mrs. A said that she grew up thinking she would not have children and had fully resolved this issue. Both her siblings had chosen not to have children, and there were no grandchildren in her family.

Mrs. A said she went into her cycle of oocyte donation expecting that she would not be successful. After learning of the triplet pregnancy, she had "a deep intuitive feeling that it was not right." She was frightened and felt like "a science experiment that went wrong." She now thought she was too old to have children, had concerns about her ability to be patient with a child, and also had financial concerns. The couple had worked very hard to put their lives in a secure financial arena. Mrs. A reported that she did not want to have her husband "work until he was 70" to support a child. Mrs. A had hoped to retire early.

In retrospect, Mrs. A felt that she had been encouraged to pursue oocyte donation by her work colleagues. Many of them had been in infertility treatment in the same clinic and, in fact, had informed her of and encouraged her to enter the Oocyte Donor Program. She regretted that her colleagues knew about her treatment, particularly that she was using donated oocytes. Although Mrs. A understood that there could be marital repercussions from her decision to terminate a pregnancy with fetuses conceived with Mr. A's sperm, she was prepared to accept these consequences. She felt that she had chosen the donor option not because she wanted it, but because her friends had encouraged her. The decision to terminate was hers alone.

Mrs. A had a D and C, which unfortunately had complications. She was hospitalized overnight and was unable to return to work for a month after her procedure. In a follow-up telephone conversation with the psychologist, Mrs. A said she felt it was "a punishment from God" for terminating the pregnancy. Nonetheless, although she had doubts, she did not regret her decision. Mr. A was not available for consultation. Mrs. A was offered counseling or a referral, which she did not accept.

Case Discussion

The unusual splitting of an embryo to produce triplets in what was initially identified as a fraternal twin pregnancy was a significant factor in Mrs. A's decision to terminate. The couple had few encounters with reproductive technology prior to their cycle, (i.e., no drug treatment, no inseminations, and no in vitro fertilization). Nothing had prepared them for this unusual occurrence.

But perhaps equally significant in Mrs. A's decision to terminate was that she had resolved issues of childlessness and had come into the program at the suggestion of colleagues. Caught up in the work environment of family-building through reproductive technologies, Mrs. A had unwittingly embarked on an "infertility adventure" that she did not fully understand or expect to succeed. All her coworkers were using their own ova in IVF treatment. They had introduced her to the possibility of oocyte donation. Mrs. A was a compliant, obedient, and hardworking woman. It is likely that there was comfort and security in being part of an "infertility group" when she entered the donor program. Until her pregnancy she did not differentiate between her ova and the donated ova. She had long ago given up the possibility of creating a family with her own genetic material. After her pregnancy, she was sorry and perhaps ashamed that other women knew of her inability to conceive with her own ova. The reality of parenting and the significant change in lifestyle it would require was not acknowledged until a positive pregnancy result was determined.

Like many other women, Mrs. A had easy, quick, and continuing access to reproductive technologies. She never went through the loss and disappointment of a miscarriage, failed IUI or IVF cycle. She had no reproductive history to test her desire to parent or her desire to become a mother. Mrs. A never thought the treatment would be successful and was unprepared for the consequences of her decision to try.

Mrs. A's religious beliefs and personal history caused her to frame her complications in the termination as a punishment from God. Not only did she endure the confusion and emotional and psychological distress of a pregnancy termination, but she also accepted medical complications, guilt, and shame as her deserved punishment.

Mrs. A and members of her family system had no history of seeking psychological support, so she was not inclined to accept our offer for therapeutic intervention or to accept a referral for therapy outside our clinic. She chose to manage her own feelings. Unfortunately, Mrs. A's husband was not a part of her decision to terminate. We have no idea what his perception or emotional state was, before or after the termination.

CASE II

Mr. and Mrs. B presented at our clinic a few weeks prior to their marriage, after a two-year relationship. Mrs. B was in her early 40s and had been adopted and raised as an only child. She knew nothing about her biological parents; her adoptive parents were both deceased. Mr. B was a successful businessman. The couple entered the Oocyte Donor Program because Mrs. B had an elevated follicle stimulating hormone (FSH) level, indicating age-related infertility. She could not pursue IVF treatment with her own ova. They had been trying to conceive for one year and had been advised that oocyte donation would give them the best chance for success.

Meeting with the couple, the reproductive endocrinologist learned that Mrs. B had undergone four terminations, the most recent four and a half years previously. Except for Mrs. B's FSH levels, all medical testing was within normal range. Prior to treatment, the couple was counseled by a psychologist affiliated with the clinic and completed psychological testing, scoring within normal range.

Mrs. B reported that, when oocyte donation was first recommended, she was upset, but at the time of the interview with the psychologist she felt more comfortable with the option. If oocyte donation was not successful, they would consider adoption. Mr. and Mrs. B requested being matched to a healthy donor with a good family medical history and some college education. They also requested that the donor be a good physical match to Mrs. B.

The couple was offered a donor match a year later. They chose to do a shared cycle, and on day three after retrieval Mrs. B had a two-embryo transfer. The day following the transfer, Mr. B called their physician expressing Mrs. B's concern about the possibility of multiples. On week eight the couple learned they had a twin pregnancy. In the early weeks of her pregnancy, Mrs. B reported severe morning sickness and discomfort with the physical changes she was experiencing.

After two normal fetal heartbeats were identified, Mrs. B was instructed to set up an appointment with an obstetrician for prenatal care. Without consultation with the infertility clinic staff, the couple decided to abort the pregnancy only days after they completed treatment in our clinic. They presented to their obstetrician and insisted on a termination. The couple was called on several occasions to discuss their decision, but they did not return the call.

Case Discussion

In Case II we do not know what precipitated the decision to terminate. The recipient couple would not return our calls. The exacerbated symptoms of a twin pregnancy may have been overwhelming for Mrs. B, affecting not only her physical comfort but also her self-confidence and self-esteem. That Mr. B called the physician right after the transfer to discuss concerns about multiples suggests that a twin pregnancy was a significant factor in the decision to terminate. We assume that their obstetrician suggested a fetal reduction to a singleton pregnancy. We do not know if the couple considered this option and rejected it.

Mrs. B had already had four previous terminations in other relationships. Perhaps it was not the twin pregnancy that was the problem, but rather the pregnancy itself, coupled with her inability or unwillingness to accept the responsibility of parenting and the lifestyle changes children require. With no information about her own genetic heritage and no living social parents, Mrs. B did not have a family system that may have helped support her in assuming a parental role. Mrs. B was in a fashion career where body image is very important. She had had two cosmetic surgeries. Perhaps the fear of the physical changes of pregnancy also played a significant factor in her decision to terminate.

We will never know why Mr. and Mrs. B aborted their pregnancy. Marital and relationship issues may have been precipitated by the pregnancy. There was a 10-year age difference between them, as well as very different educational, religious, and financial backgrounds. What we do know is that the couple's twin pregnancy was a catalyst for psychic conflict that they were unable to resolve.

CASE III

Mr. and Mrs. C, an Asian couple, had been married for more than 10 years before trying to conceive. Unsuccessful, the couple underwent two years of fertility treatment. During the treatment, Mrs. C was diagnosed with Hodgkin's disease. She underwent eight months of chemotherapy. At the time of presentation in our clinic for oocyte donation, Mrs. C had been cancer free for more than five years. She was in her early 40s.

The couple met with a reproductive endocrinologist and a staff psychologist as part of the routine consultation for oocyte donation. They completed psychological testing and scored within normal range. The psychologist reported that the couple was well informed about ooctye donation and hopeful about its success. The report cautioned, "Due to several previous traumatic experiences with medical establishments and medical staff, both are extremely sensitive and somewhat guarded in their approach and interaction with medical personnel. This should be kept in mind by clinic staff, so that they are able to undergo the donation procedure with ease." Mr. C had experienced the death of a sibling, and Mrs. C had a sibling who was mentally retarded owing to a birth injury. They also had both endured Mrs. C's diagnosis and treatment for cancer.

Mr. and Mrs. C were offered a donor 10 months after their initial presentation in the clinic. The couple learned at week eight that Mrs. C had a twin pregnancy. At this point, Mrs. C began to experience nausea and fatigue that profoundly affected her. Her past medical trauma related to cancer treatment was overpoweringly present as she went through the first trimester of her pregnancy. Overwhelmed with insecurity and fear, Mrs. C experienced such a notable degree of distress that the couple decided to abort the pregnancy. Mr. and Mrs. C made their decision without consultation with the clinic staff or affiliated psychologist. No information about their decision to terminate was available.

One year later, Mr. and Mrs. C returned to the clinic to use their frozen embryos. On a frozen cycle they achieved a singleton pregnancy and now have a healthy son.

Case Discussion

For Mrs. C, the exacerbated symptoms of a twin pregnancy provoked the memories of the stress and trauma of Mrs. C's diagnosis and treatment for cancer. We do not know if symptoms of post-traumatic stress disorder (PTSD) occurred. Mrs. C's history of growing up with a sibling who had suffered a brain injury at birth may also have made her fearful of the birthing process or fearful of having an affected child. We certainly know that Mrs. C's psychological distress, precipitated by past medical events, made it impossible for her to continue with her donor egg pregnancy.

At the time of the termination, Mrs. C began working with a psychiatrist. With therapeutic intervention, she was able to focus on her desire for a family and to have confidence to return to the clinic and to carry through a pregnancy. After a year of therapy, Mrs. C was fortunate to conceive through a frozen embryo transfer.

CONCLUSION

This chapter reports three cases in which couples who achieved a pregnancy with donated oocytes decided to terminate the pregnancy, despite the option of selective reduction and despite the fact that the embryos were the genetic offspring of the recipient husband. The couples were mature and had made a significant investment of time, money, and emotional energy in pursuing their goal of creating a family. The women had undergone intensive medical treatment. After much consideration, we do not believe we could have foreseen these unfortunate incidents or prevented them by evaluating our clients in a different way.

It is difficult to understand their complex decision to terminate pregnancy. The decision may have been precipitated by the fact of a multiple pregnancy, as reported by Marcus and Brisden (2000). Multiple gestations are associated with increased risk for mother, fetus, and newborn. Women with multiple gestation have increased symptoms of nausea and vomiting, anemia, fatigue, weight gain, heartburn, and lack of sleep (American Society for Reproductive Medicine, 2001). Multiples significantly increase financial responsibilities and may profoundly affect marital relationships. Other possible reasons for choosing to terminate have been suggested. They include lack of commitment to parenting, easy and unconsidered access to reproductive technologies, group dynamics, marital issues, body-image concerns, fear of motherhood, loss of a genetic link to the child, and medical trauma.

However, many thousands of people who have undergone reproductive treatment with donor gametes have experienced similar situations. Why did these couples interpret their condition medically and psychologically as sufficient to abort the pregnancy? Are the known reported cases just random events? If so, there is little reason for further research on the topic. Or are there many more unreported cases? Is there something more fundamental that we must learn and understand so that we can give our patients better help and counseling?

When a person has a heart operation or fights a battle with cancer, we know whether or not the medical intervention has been successful. Follow-up consultations ensure ongoing care and feedback, which will be useful in tailoring treatment for future patients. In reproductive medicine, however, there are no mechanisms in place for anything more than minimal follow-up on birth information. Clients "graduate" from the reproductive center when a pregnancy is established (usually when a fetal heart is identified). We have little insight into and very little reporting about the complex psychological processes that recipients, their spouses, families and social groups go through in the conception and parenting of offspring conceived through donor gametes. We know very little about what the children understand or experience. We do not know how complicated or unspoken feelings may tumble through future generations.

Reproductive technology has brought us to a new era of human evolution and human development. Within the last 20 years technology has enabled mature women who are beyond reproductive age to conceive with donor ova. Whereas much research has focused on the mechanics of how to make this happen, very little research has explored the psychological implications. As we lack a foundational understanding of the psychology of conception and parenting when using donor gametes, there is no real basis on which to assess and evaluate the problems of termination as we have described. We are at the dawn of an era of genetic manipulation, eventually cloning. It is imperative that we balance the technical knowledge with a deeper understanding of the related psychology. The cases we have presented are unusual and unexpected. Pregnancy termination for nonmedical reasons is certainly not a frequent occurrence in reproductive medicine. Nonetheless, the events certainly make us pause and think carefully about the treatment and opportunities that reproductive technologies provide for our clients. Offering a gift of life and a potential for a family comes with a great responsibility and is not without consequences.

Our commitment as mental health professionals to "do no harm" must include consideration of potential offspring, as well as the clients who come for counseling and consultation. The reproductive community has an immense responsibility to lay out a foundational understanding of the psychological, not only physiological, aspects of these procedures. Without this understanding, it is difficult to assess realistically the success of this technology. We can base our future only on our current understanding. In oocyte donation, we have 20 years of catching up to do.

REFERENCES

American Society for Reproductive Medicine (2001), Patient's fact sheet: Complications of multiple gestation.

Marcus, S. & Brinsden, P. (2000), Termination of pregnancy after conception with donor oocytes and donor spermatozoa. *Human Reprod.*, 15:719–722.

Part IV

Career Journeys

12

THE NURSE'S PERSPECTIVE IN A
REPRODUCTIVE PROGRAM

Maria Jackson

The growth of the nurse's role in the field of reproductive endocrinology and infertility has been wittily and accurately compared by Judith Bernstein (1991) to Topsy, the slave child in *Uncle Tom's Cabin*: unsupervised, unnurtured, and without a coherent, logical plan. This lack of discipline, she maintains, results in an outpouring of creative energy and immense productivity, which is chaotic, confused, and without direction. How the nursing role evolved from that amorphous state to the challenging, dynamic specialty that it is today is an interesting and ongoing process.

HISTORY OF INFERTILITY NURSING

In 1983, the first meeting was held to address the future of the specialty, and its focus was in two areas: credentialing and the opportunity for formal education. In 1988, the Nurses Professional Group (NPG) was added to the American Fertility Society (AFS), and today's membership numbers more than 500 nurses. The primary purpose of the NPG is nursing education. The second goal was met in 1989, when the National Association of Obstetric, Gynecologic, and Neonatal Nurses Certification Corporation (NAACOG) offered the first exam for reproductive endocrinology and infertility nursing (REIN) certification.

The nurse's role as part of a REIN team developed out of need, since the physicians could not manage all aspects of patient care, and has grown through trial and error to its current state. Bernstein describes the nontraditional aspects of this field of nursing as an attractive alternative in that it is challenging, offers nurses autonomy, provides many opportunities to learn, and is an evolving role that allows nurses to have their own patients who depend, trust and respect them for their valued contributions.

EDUCATIONAL PREPARATION

Levels of nursing education and preparedness vary greatly and affect the confidence and expertise a nurse brings to the job. Unlike other professionals in the field, for example, physicians or embryologists, there is no standardized course of study. Therefore, all nurses in this specialty have received on-the-job training that varies greatly and is totally dependent on the practice in which she works: large volume, small volume, hospital-based or private. If she finds herself in a hospital based teaching environment, she may be lucky enough to have both nurse and physician mentors and in-house educational opportunities. If her first job in the field is in a small private practice, however, opportunities to learn may be limited to her nurse colleagues, who may or more often not have the time or the talent to teach her what she needs to know. Therefore, it is not uncommon to hear a new nurse in the field say, " I hate not knowing what to do." This lack of support and knowledge can seriously undermine her confidence and may, in fact, be dangerous.

Minimum basic standards in REIN nursing have not been established, nor have learning modules been developed to assist in the training of new nurses. Moreover, there is a lack of ongoing training for experienced nurses in the specialty, unless they are allowed to attend regional or national educational meetings. According to the sponsors of one of these meetings, a large number of nurses receive no support from physicians or the practice and underwrite their own registration, travel, and lodging expenses. Furthermore, the REIN certification exam, the only standardized test that was available in this field, has been discontinued owing to lack of interest.[1]

---

[1] One can only hypothesize the reasons for this lack of interest. Without a "formal" requirement or financial incentive, taking time out of their busy lives

Finally, frequent technical advances in the field and the necessary changes inherent in these advances reinforce a sense of insecurity for both new and experienced nurses. Combined with some of the ethical challenges that frequently accompany these advances, and the lack of structured educational preparation, stress and burnout are major issues in this field of nursing.

THE NURSE'S ROLE

Defining the nurse's role is a complex task since many of her responsibilities overlap into almost all other areas of a practice. The definition also depends largely on the model of health care one espouses: medical model versus nursing model. In the medical model, the nurse's role is one of "physician extender," increasing physician productivity and decreasing the number of hours physicians work (Bernstein, 1991). The nurse role in the medical model leads to increased nursing responsibility and decreased autonomy.

By comparison, Bernstein's (1991) Independent Nurse Model views the nurse as an "independent professional" rather than as a "physician extender." By definition, the nurse's role and scope of practice is different from the physician's, yet it is just as valuable. In this model, the physician retains the role of "team captain." The patient is perceived as a complex system and his or her medical problems are part of a larger system of internal functions and social relations. The nurse's input is sought when decisions are made about patients and policies. The nurse defines her job and the extent of her responsibilities within the concept of the "team." The team validates or censures the nurse when appropriate. As a professional, however, the nurse is the best judge of her performance. The team is a forum to air conflicts, and personal ethics are

---

to study and sit for this exam may not be worth the effort. As recently as January 2003, the NPG polled the membership regarding their interest in reinstating this test. That, in my opinion, is a logical first step: however, the NPG must also educate their membership, as well as the physicians for whom they work, on the importance of this certification if they hope to have the test reinstated.

respected. Nursing research is encouraged and nursing education is supported (Bernstein, 1991).

One area of nursing practice in the REIN field that bears mentioning is the increasing use of nurse practitioners (NP). These advanced practice nurses usually have master's degrees in women's health and function as physician extenders doing everything from routine pap smears and vaginal cultures to inseminations and transvaginal ultrasounds. The NP takes a formal course of training and is licensed to perform these tests; her services, which can be billed at the same rate as the physician's, frees the physician to perform more complex procedures. From the nurse's perspective, however, financial remuneration is usually a straight salary and not based on how much she has earned for the practice.

Unlike the NP, who is licensed and certified to perform these procedures, many nurses in the field find themselves doing transvaginal ultrasounds, starting an IV, or manning PACUs (recovery rooms) without the required certifications. The performance of these procedures exposes both the nurse and the practice to liability. I do not mean to imply that nurses who perform such tasks lack skill or ability, simply the formal authority. This practice is owed largely to the broad scope of clinical responsibilities in this field and the expectation that one has to do whatever is needed. Again, regional differences (large city versus small town) and practice type (private practice versus hospital based) dictate the scope of the nurse's responsibilities.

There are some responsibilities, however, that are common to all. They include cycle management (taking the patient from initial consultation through an IVF cycle), patient education, patient support, and some degree of counseling. The nurse is the primary caregiver and the person within the practice who spends the most time with the patient. The nurse teaches the patient and her partner (if she has one) what they need to know to get them through the cycle, including the office routine, medication side effects, and injection technique. The nurse is the one who calls the patient with medication instructions and test results. These results may include such diverse variables as abnormal hormone levels, positive cultures for sexually transmitted diseases and positive pregnancy tests. When a pregnancy test goes well, the nurse is a cheerleader; when a pregnancy test result goes badly, she is a grief counselor. The nurse is the person who answers the questions patients either forgot to ask the doctor or "the silly question they didn't want to bother their doctor with." Often, she answers these questions over and over again. Unfortunately, the nurse is also the person on whom the patient takes out her frustrations, sadness, anger, hurt, and hopelessness. After a while, the strong outpouring of emotion may feel like battering.

THE SCOPE OF PRACTICE

The scope of practice and the definition of responsibilities for nurses in this field is variable. However, the following factors influence and affect the definition of nursing responsibilities: small, moderate- or large-volume practice; hospital-based versus free-standing practice; presence of REIN Fellows; the degree to which physicians interact with patients; the presence of support staff, including phlebotomists, ultrasonographers, clinical/medical assistants, psychologists, OR/PACU staff; and, finally, any satellite offices.

Approximately 30% of clinics have a counselor/psychologist/ mental health professional (MHP) on staff. In the remaining 70% of clinics, nurses commonly handle crisis intervention, grief counseling, and issues surrounding third-party reproduction, in addition to their other responsibilities (Harrington, 1999). Since the nurse is the primary caregiver, the patient or couple may perceive her as more familiar with their particular case and more approachable (and less threatening) than a formal counselor. Since discussing issues with their nurse does not require a formal appointment, patients usually perceive the nurse as more available. Patients often worry that the MHP may perceive them as "crazy" and therefore unsuitable as parents. For this reason, they are often reluctant to see the counselor even when required to do so, as in the case of sperm or ovum donation.

The role of the nurse is not only to help the couple with family building, but also to help them resolve their infertility. This role may include discussions about alternative family-building options such as adoption, egg or sperm donation, and child free living. The nurse is also a facilitator of grief, validating patient losses and supporting them through the grief process. The nurse is also a facilitator of decision making regarding treatment options and when to stop treatment (Hahn, 1991).

Counseling is not limited to psychosocial issues alone. The nurse is also an educator. Here is a partial list of the broad knowledge base that nurses practicing in this field must acquire:

- Reproductive biology
- Embryology
- Andrology: perform inseminations; sperm preps
- Ethical advisor: selective reduction; third-party reproductive choices
- Legal advisor
- Genetics
- Statistics
- Phlebotomy
- Anesthesia
- Administrative skills
- Insurance
- Ultrasonography

In the course of a day, a nurse can be a scientific advisor educating her patient in reproductive biology and embryology and discussing the results of her partner's semen analysis and its impact on their treatment options. She may be a legal advisor discussing with one couple consent forms and the contracts needed for third-party reproductive options such as egg donation or gestational carriers. She may be the referral source to an adoption agency, new obstetrician or maternal-fetal specialist. She may counsel couples on the psychosocial aspects of egg or sperm donation.[2] She may be the intermediary between an insurance company and her patient, or she may be the ethical advisor for a patient struggling with a decision to do multifetal reduction.

---

[2] An ethical dilemma I faced regarding sperm donation involved a double standard. One physician with whom I worked made it a requirement to see a counselor if a couple was pursuing ovum donation but did not require a couple to see the counselor if they were pursuing sperm donation. When confronted with this disparity, the physician adamantly refused to change the policy. Needless to say, responsibility for educating and counseling the couple pursuing sperm donation in these instances fell on the nurse, who may or not have been adequately prepared to do so.

The decision to stop or start new treatments is another area in which the nurse plays a vital role. This is especially true when couples are struggling with the decision to discontinue treatment. Physicians tend to "dangle another carrot" in front of patients when faced with multiple failed cycles. In my opinion, this tendency stems from two factors: the first is the genuine desire to give the patient what she or he wants, a pregnancy; the second is the revenue that additional cycles generate for the practice. Most times, I believe the best interests of the patient are the physician's rationale. There have, however, been some questionable decisions made on the basis that, "The patient has been counseled and chooses to proceed," or, "We don't have the right to refuse care to a patient." Clearly, there are times when we must refuse care to patients if the chances for success are so low as to make the goal untenable. As one wise MHP said to a physician after a presentation on just such issues, "Just because we have the technology to do something doesn't mean we should."

Lastly, as crass as it may seem to do so, it is important to mention the value of the nurse as a sales and marketing representative for the practice. This is especially true in large-volume practices and in cities where a patient has many choices of clinics from which to choose, each offering excellent pregnancy rates and a complete range of services. There is great competition for patients, and, if pregnancy rates are high, the rate of patients who "recycle" (if they fail to achieve pregnancy) declines significantly, making new patient referrals critical to the financial success of the practice. If "face time" with their physician is minimal, the nurse becomes the practice "ambassador" and can influence a patient's decision to stay or move on to another practice. The latter is a custom that is common in this patient population, a group that tends to "shop around."

STRESS AND BURNOUT

There are many challenges in REI nursing owing to the stress of the job. Two major problems have been identified in this specialty, high turnover and burnout. Burnout is defined by ineffectual patient interactions, primarily induced by anger and resentment due to chronic stress. Bernstein (1991) hypothesizes that erosion of the positive feelings that lead to burnout comes in three phases: the first is the *long hours and intense demands* that occur when accelerated learning is completed; the second develops after a nurse struggles to cope with the long hours, *angry patients*, emotional depletion from the number of failures, *team conflicts*, and interpersonal conflicts. Ultimately burnout is manifested in anger, resentment, and ineffectual patient interactions.

Burnout: Long Hours, Routinization of Tasks

A nurse functioning as a physician extender increases physician productivity by decreasing the number of hours physicians work. This role, however, leads to increased nursing responsibility, decreased autonomy, and, ultimately, burnout. Characteristics specific to this model of nurse as physician extender include specialization or focusing on one area of practice, thereby limiting the scope of all the others, and competition and privatization of knowledge leading to a sense of isolation. Nursing roles defined and monitored by the physician, rather than by the nurse, lead to a sense of powerlessness and anger and may lead to low self-esteem. When a nurse functions primarily as a physician extender, burnout is likely to ensue.

Powerlessness Leads to Burnout

When viewed as parts of a larger dynamic system, patients and nurses alike may be seen as robbed of power, control, and dignity. Infertility patients are often highly emotional and demanding because they are experiencing a life crisis. They are typically affluent and educated and used to being "in control" of their environment. Compounding their difficulties, the treatment options may be expensive, invasive, and painful, both emotionally and physically. Patient expectations are high, yet a successful resolution to their infertility cannot be guaranteed. According to many patients, this uncertainty makes the experience especially difficult.

The infertility experience robs patients of control, and the nurse is a convenient target for patient anger and frustration. In response, the infertility nurse may also become angry. Inasmuch as she cannot verbalize this anger, she may emotionally detach from her patients or make moral judgments about the patients' rights to reproduce. For example, "If she [the patient] can't make time in her busy schedule to come in for her testing, how will she make time to raise a child?" If there is a mental health professional (MHP) on staff, a referral for patients who are really out of control (or nurses who are out of control) is in order. If there is no MHP present, the nurse must attempt to diffuse her anger and frustrations as well as her patient's. Despite her desire to perform in an optimal manner for her patients, a sense of isolation, anger, powerlessness, and loss of self-esteem may severely affect patient care, further eroding confidence and care.

Typically, the more technology required for treatment, the greater a patient's stress, since the patient has less control than otherwise. If one were to move up the "food chain," technologically speaking, a patient doing a cycle of Clomid, with timed intercourse, generally requires much less nursing intervention than does a patient doing egg donation. Nurse burnout will be greater if the nurse practices in just one area requiring a high level of technological intervention, such as egg donation, that involves extensive contact with patients who are in the throes of anxiety, uncertainty, and powerlessness.

The daily challenge of dealing with patients' disappointments, such as negative pregnancy test results or elevated FSH (Follicle Stimulating Hormone, a predictor of ovarian potential) levels, contributes to stress and burnout because nurses often have chosen this profession because they hope to alleviate pain. According to Patricia Mahlstedt (1991), we share the same themes in our lives—hope, despair, love, hate, success, joy, failure, and sorrow. What we as clinicians have to offer others stems from our ability to experience the feelings of pain, loss, and the like in our own lives and to use these feelings in a compassionate, helping manner. Our ability to feel compassion may have determined why we chose a helping profession in the first place. Nonetheless, the wish to understand and help may contribute to our own stress. While we try to alleviate our patients' pain, which may have touched something within us, we may perceive a patient as too upset, too angry, or too demanding and we may feel we are too busy really to listen. Moreover, the way patients express their pain, (i.e., in the form of anger, criticism, or projection) may interfere with our ability to help them and may add to our stress.

Physician and Ancillary Support Staff Affect Burnout

The level of physician involvement greatly affects the nurse's role and job satisfaction. If a physician is consistently unavailable to his or her patient, the nurse is forced to "run interference" and deal with the patient's dissatisfaction. Since most of these scenarios revolve around negative outcomes, the dissatisfaction is occurring on two levels. The first dissatisfaction is the actual test results and the second is the physician's unavailability. Let us use a negative pregnancy test as an example. The dialogue might go something like this:

Nurse: "Mary, unfortunately the results of the pregnancy test were negative today. Please schedule a follow-up consultation with your physician to discuss the cycle and your treatment options."

Patient: "I don't want to wait to discuss this with my physician; I want to talk to him today. I've just spent $10,000.00 and I want answers. Do you know how hard it was to do this cycle, take all those injections and come in for all those blood tests?"

Nurses are often forced to be "on call" with no additional compensation for the intrusion; hence the feeling of working 24/7 without a break. In a high-volume practice, this may mean 20–25 calls per night. Some physicians fairly compensate nurses who take evening and weekend calls, but they are in the minority.

The presence (or absence) of support staff, such as phlebotomists, medical assistants, or Fellows, affects the day-to-day functions of a clinic and can either alleviate some of the stress or contribute to it. For example, a patient may say, "I didn't like the phlebotomist who drew my blood this morning, I have a big bruise on my arm. I want you to report her and have someone else draw my blood tomorrow."

The presence of satellite offices complicates the daily routine of patient care and certainly adds to stress. Unless the process is seamless (and despite one's best efforts it generally is not), a myriad of problems may arise. These include having to receive and interpret test results and lab values in a timely fashion from multiple locations, lost faxes, and lack of follow through for patient information. These lapses require additional phone calls to complete simple tasks. The frustration and powerlessness a nurse feels when beholden to other offices for basic information that affects treatment decisions is a reality for most nurses who have to coordinate patient care. It is not uncommon for a patient to live in one city and have monitoring done hundreds or thousands of miles away.

Opportunities for Nursing Growth Influence Burnout

To avoid burnout, nurses must be given opportunities for growth and development; they must be able to conduct research and be a vital part of the academic community. All too often, they are not given credit for the research they do conduct or are not alotted time to conduct research. Time to do research must be taken from other nursing responsibilities, and nurses are not allotted time or funds to attend national meetings or conduct independent nursing research on relevant and timely topics necessary for optimal patient care. If nurses are not given opportunities to attend national meetings to further their education, nursing research is certainly not going to be a priority. And finally, if the nurse is perceived to be an "employee," rather than a colleague, and is left out of the decision-making and conflict-resolution process, stress and burnout ensue and turnover is high.

Ethical Challenges

Challenges to one's personal ethical code are one aspect of this specialty that can leave a nurse feeling especially powerless. Whether the personal conflict involves intergenerational egg donation or multifetal reduction, our patients have the right to expect impartial treatment, and it is often difficult to separate our own values from those of the patients we treat. Ethics committees can be a voice of sanity and reason. In the absence of an ethics committee, anything can go (and sometimes does). As in most aspects of this field, we are relying on physicians to regulate themselves, since we have "guidelines" rather than laws governing the practice of reproductive medicine. A physician's views may be at odds with those of his or her staff, and, in an ideal world, open and frank discussion from all participants would be the rule rather than the commonly experienced dictum, "My way or the highway." Physicians are not challenged or stimulated to change ethically compromising practices.

Gender Influences Nursing Practice and Burnout

Any discussion on the stress and burnout associated with infertility nursing must include an understanding of who we are as women and how our gender affects change since most physicians in the field are men and most nurses are women. Bernstein (1991) describes the six factors that contribute to our sense of self, which is crucial to the level of self-esteem and sense of efficacy necessary for change. They are: (1) our gender training, which teaches us to be nurturers versus achievers and facilitators versus leaders; (2) our personality and comfort with conflict and anger; (3) our family history, which may have taught us the "hero/rescuer" role; (4) the strength of our support systems, without which change is difficult; (5) our beliefs about locus of control, that is, whether we believe control comes from within (internal) or is up to others (external); and, finally, (6) our educational preparation, which can affect our self-esteem and the respect we get.

A *New York Times* article (Corbett, 2003) addressing the current nursing shortage corroborates Bernstein's hypotheses. The author, Sara Corbett, maintains, "Historically, nurses have been portrayed as saints and sex objects . . . both dedicated and servile, treasured but not necessarily respected." She goes on to say, "Even the most positive depictions of nurses leave the impression that their work—along with their intellect—is secondary to doctors'" (p. 58). Since the role of the REI nurse is difficult to quantify, she may be especially shortchanged when it comes to accolades typically reserved for physicians.

These factors may help or hinder efforts to enact the changes needed to reduce externally induced stress in the workplace as well as internally induced stress for individual nurses. As a facilitator, rather than leader, uncomfortable with anger and conflict, the infertility nurse may not be able to effect necessary changes to prevent burnout. It is critical that each nurse know herself well enough to determine the best route to take to avoid burnout and maintain self-esteem.

Physician's Role, Team Conflict, Nurse Burnout

If one were to use Bernstein's (1991) Independent Nurse Model, in which the nurse is an "independent professional" rather than a "physician extender," the nurse's role and scope of practice would be considered to be as valuable as a physician's. The physician in this model functions as a "team captain." Unfortunately, there are far too many physicians in reproductive medicine who, knowingly or not, view themselves as gods. The physician, as a god, decides who can and should reproduce and pushes his or her staff to achieve more and possibly more patient contact, or he or she may want the staff to assume more responsibilities. In this environment, decisions are made unilaterally, and open discussion is discouraged. Only one opinion really counts. Under the guise of, "We can't refuse treatment to any patient," anything justified in the personal ethical code of the physician is considered good patient care. Given this obvious conflict of interest, the implicit rationalization becomes, in my opinion, a potential duplicitous action. For instance, medical directors routinely decide the age cut-off for potential donor egg recipients in their programs. This number varies from practice to practice and is based on the personal code of the individual physician. Each physician is refusing to treat certain patients when driven by his or her ethics. Problems arise when there is a conflict between medical director and support staff. If the medical director refuses to heed the advice and opinions of those who disagree, he or she is creating a dictatorship that empowers only one member of the (so-called) "team." It is easy to lose one's perspective when working in the high-tech world of an infertility practice. An efficient and inexpensive barometer of what is morally right or wrong is the staff, who is entrusted with the care of the program's patients.

Medicine Versus Business

I believe most physicians' primary motivation is to help their patients achieve their goal of pregnancy, and holding out hope in the form of additional cycles or different treatment options, after multiple failed cycles, can only reinforce physician omnipotence. There is, however, a practical benefit accruing to physicians when they offer more cycles, and that benefit is revenue. This specialty requires highly trained staff and state-of-the-art equipment, both of which come with a hefty price tag. Yet the potential for making money is significant despite the high overhead. Infertility, unlike other specialties, is not bound by the usual and customary reimbursements of insurance companies and HMOs. Only a few states mandate insurance coverage for infertility treatment, so many centers take no insurance and expect payment from patients before providing treatment. Unfortunately, the profits, like the accolades, are generally not distributed equitably. The nurses, who spend the most time with the patients, often benefit the least from the program's profits.

Administrators, whether in hospitals or private practices, are responsible for efficiency and cost containment. When care is determined by cost, however, conflict often follows and the patient usually suffers. In an effort to reduce costs, higher nurse-to-patient ratios often mean compromised care that dehumanizes the experience for both nurse and patient. The industry average (anecdotally) is 80–100 patients per nurse per year, a manageable number. But what happens when those numbers increase? The compromise of ideals, the inability to deliver quality care, results in guilt and powerlessness. The nurse is unable to evoke change, further undermining her self-esteem. The specialty is highly competitive. Pregnancy rates, services offered, and waiting lists for treatment or anonymous egg donors all determine patient satisfaction and referrals, the lifeblood of this field. It is therefore understandable that physicians may try to be all things to all people at the expense of their staffs.

How much does income and insurance coverage influence treatment decisions? The following example addresses both factors: if reimbursement for IVF is better than for egg donation, is it unethical to allow a patient to do repeated cycles of IVF even though she has been counseled that egg donation will statistically give much better odds? The doctor makes money and the insurance company pays so everyone is happy. Or are they? Is this arrangement really in the patient's best interest?

Is it ethical to treat same-sex couples and single women, and what if doing so violates one's personal ethical code? We are expected to respect the rights of all patients but does that same tenet apply to staff members? If our personal ethics are challenged, should we have the option to participate or not in the care of patients when that care tests the limits of our morality? I think it is safe to say that most nurses in this field are open minded and used to the cutting-edge nature of the technology. There are, however, times when even the most open-minded nurse finds her personal ethics or morals challenged. Without options, one's personal conflict or religious beliefs may be overridden by the need for a paycheck.

Finally, since this field is always on the cutting edge and continues to challenge conventional ideas of ethics and morality, I think it is imperative that all practices, small or large, hospital-based or private, be mandated to have an Ethics Committee. Opposition often comes from physicians, whose omnipotence is challenged and who rationalize that others "don't really understand what we're doing." Reproductive providers are faced with dilemmas that affect not only the couple but also their unborn child, often overlooked when decisions are made. Intergenerational egg donation is a perfect example of this irony. Not technically outside the American Society for Reproductive Medicine (ASRM) guidelines, this variation on egg donation was described by one MHP as having the "yuck factor" attached to it that makes it off limits in most clinics. To start, it challenges one of the most basic tenets of egg donor recruitment—not to coerce donors in any way. ASRM guidelines suggest that intergenerational donation is coercive because it is much more difficult for a daughter to refuse her mother who is asking for help than it would be to refuse her sister. Family relations become murky because the unborn child's sister is also his or her genetic mother and his or her mother is also his or her grandmother. How do we begin to prepare children to understand and accept this confusing lineage?

In conclusion, the field of reproductive medicine will likely continue to challenge the REI nurse on a daily basis. This is a dynamic specialty that demands a lot of the women who choose to dedicate themselves to helping build families, and the specialty has many rewards. It feels good to know that you had a part in bringing a child into this world and knowing that you made a real difference in the lives of your patients. This is especially true in the case of egg donation since the nurse is often also responsible for helping to choose an appropriate donor. Calling a patient with a positive pregnancy test is a joyful task, and sharing in the thrill of hearing the first fetal heart beats makes the not-so-pleasant aspects of the job temporarily fade.

REFERENCES

Bernstein, J. (1991), Development of the nursing role in reproductive endocrinology and infertility. In: *Principles of Infertility Nursing*, ed. C. Garner. Boca Raton, FL: CRC Press, pp. 169–178.

Corbett, S. (2003), The last shift. *The New York Times*, March 16, Section 6, p. 58.

Hahn, S. (1991), Caring for couples considering alternatives in family building. In: *Principles of Infertility Nursing*, ed. C. Garner. Boca Raton, FL: CRC Press, pp. 179–205.

Harrington, N. (1999), Evolving role of the nurse in infertility. Presented at Postgraduate Course #5, "The nurse and the infertile couple," 11th World Congress on In Vitro Fertilization and Human Reproductive Genetics, May, Sydney, Au.

Mahlstedt, P. (1991), What is essential is naked to the eye. In: *Principles of Infertility Nursing*, ed. C. Garner. Boca Raton, FL: CRC Press, pp. 157–167.

13

TWO DECADES AS AN
INFERTILITY THERAPIST

Dorothy Greenfeld

The birth of Louise Brown, the world's first "test tube baby," was reported in a letter to the editors of *The Lancet* from doctors Patrick Steptoe and Robert Edwards (1978):

> Sir,—We wish to report that one of our patients, a 30-year-old nulliparous married woman, was safely delivered by caesarean section on July 25, 1978, a normal healthy infant girl weighing 2700 g. The patient had been referred to one of us (P.C.S.) in 1976 with a history of 9 years' infertility, tubal occlusions, and unsuccessful salpingostomies done in 1970 with excision of the ampullae of both oviducts followed by persistent tubal blockages. . . . Pregnancy was established after laparoscopic recovery of an oocyte on November 10, 1977, in vitro fertilization and normal cleavage in culture media, and the reimplantation of the 8-cell embryo into the uterus 2 1/2 days later. . . . We hope to publish further medical and scientific details in your columns at a later date.

This understated report stands in stark contrast to the tumultuous worldwide reaction to its proclamation of the birth of the world's first baby conceived through in vitro fertilization. Newspapers around the globe (in contractual agreement with the *London Daily Mail*, which owned the rights to the story) announced the news that the first baby "conceived outside the womb" had been born (Greenfeld, 1978). She was named Louise Joy Brown

("Joy," according to her mother, "for the joy she brought us") (Brown, Brown, and Freeman, 1979). Her miraculous birth alerted the world to the potential, both beneficial and problematic, of assisted reproductive technology. That she was healthy and, above all, *normal*, meant that the extraordinary events surrounding her entry into the world raised the hopes of infertile couples everywhere.

At the same time, her birth set in motion a worldwide debate on the profound ethical and moral issues evoked by this new technology. Religious organizations, scientists, and commentators everywhere expressed concern about a treatment that felt "unnatural" to some and perhaps too reminiscent of the "baby production factories" in Huxley's *Brave New World* (Huxley, 1932; Biggers, 1984).

HISTORICAL BACKGROUND

Theories on reproduction were plentiful long before the advent of scientific research. For thousands of years, the common thought was that a man sowed "his seed" in a woman and it grew there "much the same way as wheat or barley seed" (Lazzaro, 1979). On the other hand, 17th- and 18th-century biologists believed that the woman's egg contained the embryo in a preformed state. An early theory postulated that if the egg were exposed to the "vapors from the semen," the so-called *aura spermatica*, fertilization would occur. Long before Steptoe and Edwards began their fateful collaboration, researchers had been considering the possibilities of in vitro fertilization. In fact, the original push for IVF did not come from the medical establishment. Edwards was a biologist, an animal researcher "who understood and appreciated the similarity in biology between humans and other mammals" (Silver, 1997). Much of the early success in reproductive science, and, indeed, much of the work today, is accomplished through research on animals.

In 1779, an Italian physiologist, Lazzaro Spallanzani, used frogs and toads to demonstrate that physical contact between the egg and seminal fluid was necessary for the egg to develop. By showing that the frog semen he collected could cause unfertilized frog eggs to develop into tadpoles, Spallanzani was the first to achieve artificial insemination in the laboratory under controlled conditions. In 1782, to show that the process could be repeated with mammals, he successfully inseminated a cocker spaniel. He described this achievement:

> Sixty-two days after the injection of the seed, the bitch brought forth three lively whelps, two male and one female, resembling in color and shape not the bitch only, but the dog also from which the seed had been taken. Thus did I succeed in fecundating this quadruped: and I can truly say, that I never received greater pleasure upon any occasion, since I first cultivated experimental philosophy [Betteridge, 1981].

Another early contributor to the science of reproductive technology was John Hunter, a Scottish physician and surgeon to King George III. In 1790, Dr. Hunter met a couple who were infertile as a result of the husband's hypospadia, a malformation of the penis which left him unable to impregnate his wife. Dr. Hunter told the man to collect the semen in a "warm cup" and to inject the fluid into his wife's vagina using a syringe. Although this was the first human pregnancy achieved through artificial insemination, Hunter never reported his accomplishment for fear of public outcry that he had encouraged the "unnatural act" of masturbation. Long after Hunter's death, his cousin reported the feat in a paper he was writing about hermaphroditic dogs (Gosden, 1999).

A century later, in 1891, Walter Heape accomplished the first successful embryo transfer. Heape demonstrated that fertilized ova could be flushed from a rabbit's fallopian tubes and transferred to a surrogate mother. Whether he transferred embryos from pigmented rabbits to the uteri of albino rabbits, or vice versa, he noted that "the litters always bred true to the donors rather than the hosts" (Gosden, 1999). After mating two Angora rabbits, he transferred the embryos to the uterus of a Belgian hare. Thus, the Belgian hare "represents the first mammal ever to have given birth to offspring that was not genetically her own" (Silver, 1997).

The partnership between Patrick Steptoe, a gynecologist in practice in a small town in the north of England, and Robert Edwards, a biologist at Cambridge University, came late in their careers.

Edwards earned his Ph.D. in Animal Genomics by artificially inseminating mice and observing the development of mouse embryos. In 1960, close friends of his became infertile as a result of the wife's blocked fallopian tubes. Edwards wondered "what would happen if you were able to remove an egg from the ovary, fertilize and put it back into the womb," in effect bypassing the blocked tubes (Edwards and Steptoe, 1982). He soon began work on the maturation of human oocytes in vitro. On occasion, he was able to obtain human eggs from surgical patients having parts of their ovaries removed, but these were hard to come by. Sheep and pig ovaries were easy to get from slaughterhouses, and he sometimes received monkey ovaries from labs. This work led to the observation on the differences in oocyte maturation time of each species: mice, brief; sheep, cows, and monkeys, intermediate; humans and pigs, long (Edwards, 1965).

Edwards now knew how to achieve fertilization in vitro in humans but still faced the question of how best to remove the eggs. At this propitious time, Patrick Steptoe began working on a textbook describing the use of laparoscopy in gynecology. Like Edwards's, Steptoe's work had been inspired, in part, by the quandary of infertility. He described how deeply moved he had been as a medical student when sitting in on a conference between a surgeon and a patient with blocked fallopian tubes when the surgeon told the woman she would never bear children (Edwards and Steptoe, 1982).

Throughout his career in gynecology, Steptoe had been struggling with the problem of blocked fallopian tubes and other aspects of infertility. One of the things that irked him was that exploratory surgery was achievable only with a laparotomy, which was major, quite debilitating surgery. Subsequently, he read about the work of a French physician, Raoul Palmer, who had developed a laparoscope. This original model was difficult to maneuver. It was filled with a balloon of carbon dioxide and inserted into the abdominal cavity, where it was used like a telescope. Attached to it was an electric lamp that heated up so quickly that the surgeon had to work rapidly or the lamp would overheat and break.

When German physician Hans Frangenheim developed a better model, Steptoe talked his department into buying one. On his lunch hour he would go to the mortuary and practice laparoscopies on cadavers; he eventually performed over 126 of these procedures on cadavers to perfect his technique. In 1964, he attended a symposium on gynecological laparoscopy in Palermo, where he met Palmer, who reported that he wanted to perform sterilization through the laparoscope but was not permitted to do so in Catholic France. Frangenheim reported the same resistance from Catholics in Germany. As a result, they asked Steptoe to pioneer the procedure in England. Steptoe went on to perform the first 50 cases of sterilization through the laparoscope. "Palmer introduced us to laparoscopy; Frangenheim developed the instrumentation, but Steptoe taught us how to use it" (Edwards and Steptoe, 1982).

Steptoe and Edwards began their collaborative work in 1968. Their aim was to improve the process of fertilization outside the womb. After studying embryos growing in culture and being assured that they developed normally, the researchers began the process of embryo transfer. They worked together for almost a decade before finally achieving a pregnancy. The first patient had an ectopic pregnancy, and the second patient who became pregnant miscarried within a couple of weeks.

Since the birth of Louise Brown, thousands of children have been born as a result of this treatment. The first baby conceived through IVF in the United States was born in 1985, followed by another 337 babies reported in that year. By 1993, the number had jumped to 6870. In 1999, 21,904 deliveries resulted in the birth of 30,967 infants in the United States alone. Of these, 13,909 were singletons, 6971 were twins, 980 were triplets, and 44 were deliveries of higher order than triplet (Greenfeld, 2002). IVF, developed initially to treat women with blocked fallopian tubes, rapidly became the method of treatment for a variety of infertility diagnoses, including endometriosis, anovulation, and male infertility. Within a very few years following the birth of Louise Brown, the development of embryo cryopreservation, egg donation, gestational surrogacy and the increased incidence of multiple gestation transformed the landscape of infertility treatment in dramatic and unprecedented ways.

IVF DURING THE 1980S

In 1982, Yale became one of six programs in the United States to offer IVF. I had just graduated from social work school with a keen interest in women's health issues. It was my good fortune to be hired to work in the infertility clinic immediately after the first IVF baby was born at Yale. My role was to serve as "gatekeeper" in a program where an innovative new treatment had caused great concern in the community. At the time, clinicians were fearful that emotionally unstable patients might stir up unwelcome controversy for the program, so my role initially was to evaluate potential patients for "suitability" and "emotional stability." It was by no means clear who was "unsuitable for treatment," but it made sense that some sort of screening was prudent for keeping a lid on things, and my job was to figure out how to do that effectively.

It is difficult for me to describe my feelings in the early years of this work. Breathtaking comes to mind. I was at once terrified and excited—terrified by being a new clinician dealing with the unfamiliar and unknown and struggling with a sense of my ignorance and incompetence (surely they can see that I don't know what I'm doing), yet excited and stimulated to be part of a pioneering new enterprise. I was completely unprepared for the intensity of the emotional struggles of the women I was trying to help, and often I was overwhelmed by a sense of guilt (at being so lucky with regard to my own fertility), ignorance, and fear that I could not possibly help. I lived in terror of those times when patients inevitably asked me, "Do you have children?" My standard response, "I'm happy to answer that question, but could we talk about what it means to you?" felt like a cowardly way of deflecting their implied "How can you possibly understand what I am going through?" Interestingly, now that I am past the reproductive years (at least the natural reproductive years, and not those recently redefined by egg donation), I am no longer asked that question.

Fortunately, it was not all scary. It was also very exciting to be on the frontier of a new medical breakthrough, to be the first to address new and challenging problems and to help people who could not be helped otherwise. Those of us who were among the first mental health professionals working in IVF were defining our roles as we met with patients going through the procedure.

From those first patients I learned the basics of counsel and support for infertile couples going through IVF. This educative process had a very strong impact on me because, as I learned about the process, I was simultaneously learning about how to educate patients about the process—specifically about ovarian stimulation, oocyte retrieval, mixing of egg and sperm in vitro, and embryo transfer. These terms are now a familiar part of the language of the infertile and are crucial to the discourse between patients and their clinicians, but then they were new to everyone and careful educational efforts were crucial to helping patients understand what they were undertaking. At the time, there was much debate among members of the mental health profession about how best to define our role. Those of us who were learning about this process wrote about our experiences in an attempt to help shape and influence the evolution of our role.

In those early days, the technology was more primitive than now. Oocyte retrieval was accomplished by means of laparoscopy, meaning that the woman had to undergo general anesthesia and surgery in order to have her eggs retrieved. Her husband, in the meantime, while his wife was taken to the recovery room, was handed a cup and directed to the men's room in the hospital to obtain the specimen. (On those rare occasions that the husband was unable to produce a sample, general mayhem ensued. There was the woman just recovering from anesthesia, waking up to learn that the 20 eggs she had produced would not be fertilized because her husband was not able to do his part.) The early years of IVF treatment did not include embryo cryopreservation, so any eggs obtained by the women were mixed with the semen of her partner and the couple was faced with the decision of whether to transfer all embryos or to have some destroyed. As a result, the increased numbers of multiple gestations led to the development of yet another procedure, multifetal pregnancy reduction.

In the beginning, we learned a great deal about the emotional turmoil and resiliency of patients undergoing IVF. We learned that it can be frightening for patients, that the euphoria and dysphoria they experience are part of the process, an emotional turbulence that echoes the suffering accompanying years of infertility. The question of whether or not she will actually produce eggs, the question of whether or not the eggs will fertilize, and then the question of whether or not the embryos will implant—all cause a great deal of apprehension for patients already concerned about their anxiety levels. They worry, "Am I going crazy, and will the craziness I feel prevent me from getting pregnant?" At the same time, others are usually telling them that they should keep a positive attitude, the implication being that an upbeat and relaxed mental attitude will by itself make pregnancy possible. Therapists learned early on that normalizing the process, "Yes, it feels crazy," "No, you are not crazy," "How could you not be grieving?" was the best way to decrease these anxiety levels.

Lorna and Walter K began trying to conceive immediately after getting married, because, as Lorna said, "I couldn't wait to be a mother." When she failed to conceive right away, she relied on the advice of their family doctor, who recommended daily temperature monitoring and timed intercourse. After several years of these procedures, the couple sought a consultation with a renowned fertility specialist in Boston who performed a laparoscopy and determined that Lorna had blocked fallopian tubes. Lorna described the devastating feelings that followed the diagnosis. At that time it meant that, for all practical purposes, she could never have children. The mystery of how her tubes became blocked added to her guilt and anguish: was it the abortion she had at age 15? the promiscuity in her early 20s? or was it the appendectomy she had at age 19?

What followed for her was a time of mourning, but also some relief at having a name for the problem and an end to constantly thinking, month after month, that "this cycle could be the one." The Ks had been married for 10 years at the time of our meeting. They had traveled from a small town in northern Maine to our program, at that time the nearest center to offer IVF. Lorna described many years of mourning the loss of having her "own children," but at the time of our meeting the couple was actively pursuing adoption. She explained that, once IVF was made possible, they felt it was worth a try. They observed that "we don't want to find ourselves years later saying that we wished we had tried but didn't." Since the Ks did not become pregnant, I learned from this couple that the technology, while offering great hope, also offered a kind of closure. Before IVF treatment, "the end of the line" was hard to define. Now that this treatment was available, couples could take advantage of the possibilities the treatment offered and simultaneously put the issue to rest and move on.

FROZEN EMBRYOS

IVF treatment was greatly enhanced by the development of cryo-preservation of embryos. Animal research, once again, was in the forefront when the first successful freezing and thawing of embryos was accomplished in mice in 1971. Shortly afterward, this success was repeated in cows, rabbits, sheep, and goats (Wilmut and Rowson, 1973). The first human born as a result of embryo cryo-preservation was Zoe Leyland, born in Australia in 1984.

Since that success, cryopreservation has been both a blessing and a curse to IVF treatment centers around the world. The bless-ings are many. Prior to freezing, all embryos were either implanted into the uterus or discarded. Preserving embryos through freez-ing makes it possible for patients to have more than one treatment cycle from a single egg retrieval procedure. Another great advan-tage to cryopreservation of embryos is that it makes it possible for patients to preserve embryos for possible future use. Embryo cryo-preservation has also been a curse for centers with extra, discarded, and "abandoned" embryos filling ranks of clinics around the world and raising ethical concerns about their ultimate disposition (Klock et al., 2001).

A well-documented, very complicated example of the latter hap-pened in 1981, when the Rios, a couple from Los Angeles, went through IVF treatment in Melbourne. Mrs. R produced three eggs, with one embryo transferred and two frozen. She became preg-nant but miscarried within a few weeks. Feeling very upset and not ready to try again, the Rios went home to California and left the frozen embryos in Australia. In 1983, they were killed in a plane crash while traveling in Chile. It was soon determined that the Rios had left behind an estate worth eight million dollars, without heirs or a will. When newspapers learned about the "abandoned embryos," women from all over the world volunteered to be a sur-rogate mother of the potential heir. Much debate, litigation, and confusion ensued about the appropriate disposition of the embryos (Gosden, 1999).

In my own work, I noticed that frozen embryos meant that cou-ples now had a great deal more to say about the number of embryos transferred, and for many that was a great relief. For others, however, the ethical dilemmas raised by the question of "embryo disposition" (that is, whether to freeze, discard, or donate the embryos for research) caused great anxiety. I also noted that couples often initially develop strong feelings of attachment for the embryos, but that these feelings may change over time (hence, the numbers of "abandoned embryos" in clinic freezers around the world).

In addition, as the Rios' case demonstrates, there are complex issues raised by the death of one or both of the partners. Similarly, disposition may be contested if the partners divorce, raising questions about embryo custody that must be considered prior to IVF at a time when a couple may not want to contemplate such outcomes.

THE ADVENT OF "THIRD-PARTY REPRODUCTION"

The first baby born as a result of oocyte donation was in 1983 in Australia. The case involved a 29-year-old patient who, while going through an IVF cycle, donated one of her eggs to a 25-year-old woman with premature ovarian failure (Lutjen, Trounson, and Leeton, 1984). While the original effort was to treat a particularly devastating diagnosis for young women, egg donation has become a treatment for women with a variety of diagnoses, including repeated failed cycles of IVF, genetic disorders, recurring pregnancy loss, and advanced reproductive age. In the early years of oocyte donation, eggs were retrieved through the laparoscope, a surgical procedure requiring anesthesia. For that reason, women already scheduled for that procedure—tubal ligation patients and women going through IVF—were thought to be ideal candidates. However, the number of tubal ligation patients willing to donate eggs was limited, and the number of IVF patients willing to donate their "extra eggs" dwindled with the advent of embryo cryopreservation.

The landscape changed considerably once egg retrieval with ultrasound became the norm. Programs actively began to recruit and compensate donors. The idea was that donors should be compensated fairly but not overpaid, for fear that excessive payment would effectively coerce donation from women who might not be psychologically prepared to donate.

Currently, the issue of compensation for donors remains controversial. This controversy was brought home in 1999, when a couple placed an ad in the school newspapers of several Ivy League colleges seeking "a tall, attractive and very bright young woman with high SAT scores" to donate. The compensation fee offered was $50,000. While this was clearly an exorbitant amount, the definition of "excessive compensation" has changed considerably over time. Compensation from many programs is now more than $5000, and many private recruiters seek substantially more, depending on the qualifications of the donor (Marshall et al., 1999).

Shortly after our egg donation program started, I was asked to take an active role in the recruitment, screening, and matching of donors. I was not the donor recruiter, exactly, but as a member of the team, took part in the process. Initially, I found myself looking at women in a new way: who would make a good donor? At the same time, I had to deal with protective feelings about these young women. I struggled with thoughts like, "If you were my daughter I wouldn't want to see you getting yourself into this, taking these risks with your body for money." Sometimes, I would screen a donor and think, "What a great match she would make for Mrs. X," and then I'd be shocked at how easy it is to feel a Godlike sense of power over matters of such basic importance. The screening process itself, by comparison, was relatively simple.

The "Host Uterus": Gestational Surrogacy

Prior to IVF, surrogacy generally involved a scenario where the surrogate was artificially inseminated with the sperm of the husband of the infertile woman. After the birth, the baby would be released to the couple (Hanafin, 1999). This process came into practice in the 1970s, and by the 1980s there were three centers offering the process of screening and matching surrogates to infertile couples. But the advent of IVF greatly changed the picture of surrogacy when, in 1987, a woman gave birth to a baby not genetically related to her through the process of a successful embryo transfer and IVF. (Interestingly, Steptoe and Edwards had attempted this procedure a few years—to a great hue and cry—but the treatment was unsuccessful.) Subsequently, gestational surrogacy, or the use of a "host uterus," has become, if not routine, at least an accepted method of treatment in many IVF treatment centers around the country.

Because there is no central registry documenting these arrangements, it is difficult to ascertain the number of successes. One study in 1997 reported that there were approximately 6000 births through surrogacy, and 500 of such pregnancies were through the use of gestational surrogacy and IVF (Hanafin, 1999). This treatment has not been without its controversies and some well-known legal battles. However, early concerns about a surrogate who would be unable to give up a baby she had been carrying for nine months, or about wealthy couples who would use carriers to avoid the burdens of pregnancy, have proven largely unfounded. What is clear is that women without a functioning uterus who may have spent many years thinking that they would never be mothers, now can have children through the use of a gestational surrogate. In addition, gestational surrogacy has opened up heretofore unimagined possibilities. For example, it has made it possible for mothers to carry pregnancies for their infertile daughters. It has made it possible for two gay men to have children—often through the use of an egg donor and a surrogate, with the resulting child related to one of the couple through artificial insemination.

MULTIPLE PREGNANCY AND MULTIFETAL PREGNANCY REDUCTION

Another dramatic consequence of IVF and assisted reproductive technology is the increased number of multiple pregnancies and increased numbers of twins, triplets, and other higher order multiples. For example, in the United States, during the period from 1972–1974 to 1989, the rate per 100,000 live births of higher order multiples born to Caucasian women increased threefold, from 29.2 to 85 per 100,000 births (Luke, 1994). In fact, 48% of the 12,327 infants delivered through some sort of assisted reproductive technology in 1990–1991 were from multiple gestations (Wilcox et al., 1996).

In the early years of assisted reproductive technology, uncontrolled ovarian stimulation and lack of ultrasound monitoring were more commonly the causes of this epidemic than was IVF treatment. However, the advent of ultrasound and the ability to limit the number of embryos transferred did not, in fact, limit the number of embryos transferred, and the problem actually increased in

IVF programs during the 1990s. The reasons are largely economic: IVF programs need to maximize their success rates in order to get more patients, and the best way to maximize their success rates is to implant more than one embryo, thus significantly raising the chances for multiple pregnancy.

Part of the controversy surrounding the increased numbers of multiple pregnancies and multiple births has to do with pregnancy outcome. Most studies indicate that IVF children are generally normal and without developmental problems. When problems do occur, however, they are generally a result of low birth weight and premature delivery, often a consequence of multiple pregnancy. In fact, higher order multiple pregnancies represent the largest single cause of poor obstetrical outcome and neonatal difficulties (Veeck, Davis, and Rosenwaks, 2001). Ironically, the treatment offered to improve the outcome of multiple pregnancy is achieved through multifetal pregnancy reduction—reducing a triplet pregnancy to a twin pregnancy with the intent of giving the twins a better chance for a healthy outcome, for example. In the 1990s, more and more couples were being offered pregnancy reduction as a way of insuring the health of the surviving fetus(es).

CONCLUSION

Within a very few years following the birth of Louise Brown, the development of embryo cryopreservation, egg donation, gestational surrogacy, and the increased incidence of multiple gestation had a dramatic impact on reproductive medicine. The future promises to be no less remarkable. With the increased use of preimplantation genetic diagnosis and molecular genetics, IVF treatment will select the best embryos for optimum success rates while eliminating most genetically transmitted disease. According to Silver, "What IVF does inherently is to provide access to the egg and the embryo—and with that access, it becomes possible to observe and modify the embryo and its genetic material" (Lazzaro, 1979). Modifying the embryo and its genetic material is only the most controversial of the many possibilities created by IVF technology.

REFERENCES

Betteridge, K. (1981), An historical look at embryo transfer. *J. Reprod. Fertil.*, 62:1–13.

Biggers, J. D. (1984), In vitro fertilization and embryo transfer in historical perspective. In: *In Vitro Fertilization and Embryo Transfer*, ed. A. Trounson & C. Wood. London: Churchill & Livingstone, pp. 3–15.

Brown, L., Brown, J. & Freeman, S. (1979), *Our Miracle Called Louise: A Parents' Story*. London: Paddington Press.

Edwards, R. (1965), Maturation in vitro of mouse, sheep, cow, pig, rhesus monkey and human ovarian oocytes. *Nature*, 308:349–351.

———— & Steptoe, P. (1982), *A Matter of Life*. London: Sphere.

Gosden, R. (1999), *Designing Babies: The Brave New World of Reproductive Technology*. New York: Freeman.

Greenfeld, D. (1978), *London Daily Mail*, July 25.

———— (2002), Assisted reproductive technology in the United States: 1999 results generated from the American Society of Reproductive Medicine/ Society for Assisted Reproductive Technology registry. *Fertil. Steril.*, 78:918–931.

Hanafin, H. (1999), Surrogacy and gestational carrier participants. In: *Infertility Counseling: A Comprehensive Handbook for Clinicians*, ed. L. H. Burns & S. N. Covington. New York: Parthenon.

Huxley, A. (1932), *Brave New World*. London: Chatto & Windus.

Klock, S., Sheinin, S. & Kazer, R. (2001), The disposition of unused frozen embryos. *N. Engl. J. Med.*, 365:68–69.

Lazzaro, T. (1979), Spallanzani's seminal discovery. *New Scientist*.

Luke, B. (1994), The changing pattern of multiple births in the United States: Maternal and infant characteristics, 1973 and 1990. *Obstet. Gynecol.*, 84:101–6.

Lutjen, P., Trounson, A. & Leeton, J. (1984), The establishment and maintenance of pregnancy using in vitro fertilization and embryo donation in a patient with primary ovarian failure. *Nature*, 307:174.

Marshall, L., Emrich, J., Hjelm, M., Shandell, A. & Letterie, G. (1999), What motivates paid ovum donors? In: *Towards Reproductive Certainty*, ed. R. Jansen & D. Mortimer. New York: Parthenon.

Silver, L. (1997), *Remaking Eden: Cloning and Beyond in a Brave New World*. New York: Avon Books.

Steptoe, P. & Edwards, R. (1978), Birth after the reimplantation of a human embryo. *Lancet*, 2:366.

Veeck, L., Davis, O. & Rosenwaks, Z. (2001), Avoiding multiple pregnancy after assisted reproductive technologies. In: *Iatrogenic Multiple Pregnancy: Clinical Implications*, ed. I. Blickstein & L. Keith. New York: Parthenon.

Wilcox, L., Kiely, J. & Melvin, C. (1996), Assisted reproductive technologies: Estimates of their contribution to multiple births and newborn hospital stays in the United States. *Fertil. Steril.*, 65:361–366.

Wilmut, I. & Rowson, L. (1973), The successful low temperature preservation of mouse and cow embryos. *J. Reprod. Fertil.*, 33:352–353.

AUTHOR INDEX

CONTENTS